FATTY LIVER RECIPES COOKBOOK

Essential Guide to Reversing Fatty Liver Disease with 100+ Simple, Healthy Meals.

DONNA M. ROTH

CONTENTS

INTRODUCTION

We would like to take this opportunity to welcome you to the "Fatty Liver Recipe Cookbook," where the path to improved liver health starts with the preparation of delectable dishes. When we live in a society where our lifestyle choices often put our health at risk, it is essential that we have a solid awareness of the influence that nutrition has on liver function. The illness known as fatty liver, which is defined by the accumulation of extra fat in the cells of the liver, requires care and a proactive approach to diet due to its severity.

When you use this cookbook as a guide, you will be able to create meals that not only excite your taste senses but also aid in the repair of your liver. In this culinary journey, we will explore meals that are specifically designed to enhance liver health. These recipes will make use of foods that are well-known for their nourishing and healing capabilities.

In the introduction, the complexities of fatty liver are discussed in depth, with an emphasis on the origins, symptoms, and risk factors associated with the condition. We give a complete overview of the fundamentals of nutrition and highlight the relevance of maintaining a balanced diet in minimizing the consequences of this illness. In this course, you will learn about the function of macronutrients and micronutrients, as well as practical dietary advice that are specifically designed for those who are struggling with fatty liver disease.

The core of this cookbook resides in its selection of dishes meant to not only please your appetite but also contribute to the well-being of your liver. Every single dish is a demonstration of how taste and nutrition can be harmoniously combined. From nourishing breakfast treats to delicious lunch and dinner alternatives, as well as snacks, appetizers, and desserts that are designed with a healthy twist, and everything in between.

For the purpose of making your trip even more accessible, we provide carefully selected meal plans that are flexible enough to accommodate a variety of requirements and preferences about food. Whether you're a culinary newbie or a seasoned chef, these dishes are developed with simplicity and accessibility in mind, guaranteeing that everyone can start on this culinary path toward greater liver health.

As you walk through the pages of the "Fatty Liver Recipe Cookbook," consider it not simply a culinary guide but a companion in your search for a better, happier life. Let the scents, textures, and tastes of these dishes bring in a new chapter of energy and well-being. Welcome to a culinary experience where sustaining your body takes center stage, one tasty cuisine at a time.

UNDERSTANDING FATTY LIVER

Fatty liver, a frequent health problem in our contemporary lives, is a disorder defined by the buildup of excess fat inside liver cells. This introduction chapter tries to untangle the complexity of fatty liver, giving a complete overview to equip readers with information about this widespread ailment.

Delving into the causes and risk factors, we study how lifestyle choices, nutrition, obesity, and metabolic variables contribute to the development of fatty liver. Understanding these underlying variables is crucial in implementing preventative measures and making educated decisions for a healthy liver.

Symptoms and diagnosis are key components of our investigation, offering insight on how fatty liver appears and the diagnostic approaches applied by healthcare experts. By identifying the indicators early on, people may take proactive efforts towards controlling their liver health.

As we continue on the path of studying fatty liver, this chapter provides as a basis for the remaining portions of the cookbook. It highlights the significance of awareness and proactive steps, setting the scene for the gastronomic adventure that follows in the search for a healthy liver and general well-being.

IMPORTANCE OF A HEALTHY DIET

A balanced diet is a cornerstone in the treatment and prevention of fatty liver, playing a crucial role in supporting liver health and general well-being. This section addresses the substantial influence that dietary choices may have on alleviating the consequences of fatty liver, giving insights into why a conscientious approach to nutrition is crucial.

1. **Managing Fat Intake:** Controlling the kind and quantity of lipids ingested is key in resolving fatty liver. Emphasizing good fats such as those found in avocados, almonds, and olive oil while limiting saturated and Tran's fats leads to a balanced and liver-friendly diet.

2. **Balancing Macronutrients:** Striking a balance among macronutrients—proteins, carbs, and fats—supports general health. A diet rich in lean proteins, whole grains, and fruits and vegetables delivers critical nutrients without overburdening the liver.

3. **Controlling Sugar and Processed Foods:** Excessive sugar consumption and highly processed diets might lead to liver fat formation. Understanding the effect of added sugars and processed carbs helps people to make decisions that promote liver function.

4. **Embracing Antioxidant-Rich Foods:** Antioxidants have a critical role in fighting inflammation and oxidative stress, both of which are related with fatty liver. Including fruits, vegetables, and other antioxidant-rich foods in the diet promotes liver function and decreases inflammation.

5. **Moderating Alcohol Consumption:** For patients with alcoholic fatty liver disease, moderation or abstinence from alcohol is crucial. Even with non-alcoholic fatty liver disease, reducing alcohol consumption is suggested to preserve overall liver health.

6. **Hydration and Herbal Teas:** Staying well-hydrated promotes liver function. Herbal teas, such as dandelion or green tea, are renowned for their ability to enhance liver function and may be added into a balanced diet.

Understanding the symbiotic link between a balanced diet and liver health allows people to make educated decisions that contribute to the prevention and treatment of fatty liver. By adopting a mindful attitude to diet, people may begin on a path towards a better, happier existence.

CAUSES AND RISK FACTORS OF FATTY LIVER

Fatty liver is a complicated disorder impacted by a mix of lifestyle, genetic, and metabolic factors. Understanding the causes and risk factors is crucial in navigating the intricacies of this disorder. This section gives light on the important factors to the development of fatty liver.

- ❖ **Poor Dietary Choices:** Consuming a diet heavy in saturated fats, Tran's fats, and sweets may lead to a buildup of fat in the liver. Processed meals, sugary drinks, and high caloric intake add greatly to the risk of fatty liver.

- ❖ **Obesity and Overweight:** Excess body weight, especially around the abdomen region, is a substantial risk factor for fatty liver. Obesity is intimately connected to insulin resistance, which plays a role in the formation of fat in liver cells.

- ❖ **Insulin Resistance and Type 2 Diabetes:** Insulin resistance, typically related with obesity, is a condition where the body's cells do not react properly to insulin. This metabolic imbalance adds to fat storage in the liver, raising the risk of fatty liver disease. Type 2 diabetes, strongly connected to insulin resistance, is also a risk factor.

- ❖ **Genetics:** Genetic factors may predispose people to fatty liver. Some individuals may be more prone to acquiring the illness owing to hereditary features that impact how their body processes and retains fat.

- ❖ **Metabolic Syndrome:** Fatty liver is a component of metabolic syndrome, a cluster of disorders that includes high blood pressure, elevated cholesterol levels, insulin resistance, and obesity. The interaction of these variables adds to the development of fatty liver.

- ❖ **Rapid Weight reduction:** Quick and rapid weight reduction, particularly via crash diets or certain medical procedures, may prompt the release of stored fat into the circulation, leading to its buildup in the liver.

- ❖ **Excessive Alcohol Consumption:** While typically linked with alcoholic fatty liver disease, excessive alcohol use is also a risk factor for non-alcoholic fatty liver disease. Alcohol adds to liver inflammation and may aggravate existing liver disorders.

- ❖ **Age and Hormonal Changes:** Fatty liver seems to be more frequent in middle-aged and older persons. Hormonal changes, such as those happening after menopause, May also impact fat distribution and metabolism, raising the risk.

By recognizing these causes and risk factors, people may take proactive efforts toward avoiding and controlling fatty liver, increasing overall liver health and well-being.

SYMPTOMS AND DIAGNOSIS OF FATTY LIVER

Fatty liver sometimes develops quietly, with minor symptoms or, in rare situations, none at all. This section discusses the signs of fatty liver and the diagnostic tools performed to diagnose and evaluate the illness.

SYMPTOMS:

- **Fatigue:** Individuals with fatty liver may suffer prolonged weariness, which might be due to the pressure on the liver as it processes fat.

- **Abdominal Discomfort:** Some may report soreness or a sensation of weight in the upper right side of the abdomen, where the liver is situated.

- **Elevated Liver Enzymes:** Blood tests may demonstrate high liver enzyme levels, suggesting liver inflammation. However, some persons with fatty liver may have normal enzyme levels.

- **Weakness:** General weakness and a sensation of malaise may be evident, indicating the influence of fatty liver on general health.

- **Unexplained Weight Loss:** In certain situations, persons with fatty liver may have unexplained weight loss, especially if the illness evolves to a more severe state.

DIAGNOSIS:

- **Blood Tests:** Liver function tests evaluate the levels of enzymes and other chemicals in the blood, giving a first indication of liver health.

- **Imaging Studies:** Non-invasive imaging methods, such as ultrasonography, CT scans, or MRI, may see the liver and identify the presence of extra fat.

- **Liver Biopsy:** In some circumstances, a liver biopsy may be needed to examine the degree of liver damage. This entails extracting a tiny tissue sample from the liver for microscopic examination.

- **Fibro Scan or Transient Elastography:** This imaging method examines hepatic stiffness, giving information on fibrosis or scarring in the liver.

- **Clinical Assessment:** Healthcare practitioners assess criteria such as medical history, risk factors, and physical tests to determine the possibility of fatty liver

NUTRITION ESSENTIAL NEEDED

Understanding the impact of macronutrients and micronutrients is crucial in constructing a diet that promotes liver health, especially in the setting of fatty liver. This section addresses the role of these vital nutrients in fostering general well-being.

Macronutrients:

1. **Proteins:** Adequate protein consumption is necessary for liver function, since it stimulates tissue regeneration and helps prevent muscle loss. Lean protein sources such as chicken, fish, tofu, and lentils are favored to lessen the stress on the liver.

2. **Carbohydrates:** Opting for complex carbs like whole grains, fruits, and vegetables gives a consistent stream of energy and fiber. This may help manage blood sugar levels and contribute to a balanced diet.

3. **Fats:** Choosing healthy fats, such as those found in avocados, almonds, and olive oil, is vital. Limiting saturated and Trans fats helps regulate cholesterol levels and minimizes the danger of additional fat formation in the liver.

Micronutrients:

1. **Vitamins:**
   Vitamin E: An antioxidant that may help decrease liver inflammation. Sources include nuts, seeds, spinach, and broccoli.
   Vitamin C: Supports the immune system and may assist in lowering oxidative stress. Found in citrus fruits, berries, and bell peppers.

2. **Minerals:**
   Selenium: Acts as an antioxidant and is found in Brazil nuts, shellfish, and whole grains.
   Zinc: Supports immunological function and wound healing, with sources including meat, dairy, and legumes.

3. **Other Nutrients:**
   Omega-3 Fatty Acids: Found in fatty fish, flaxseeds, and walnuts, they may have anti-inflammatory properties and improve general cardiovascular health.
   Choline: Important for liver function and found in eggs, lean meats, and cruciferous vegetables.

Maintaining a well-balanced and nutrient-dense diet is crucial in treating fatty liver. Monitoring the consumption of these macronutrients and micronutrients not only improves liver health but also adds to overall metabolic well-being.

DIETARY GUIDELINES FOR FATTY LIVER DIETARY GUIDELINES FOR FATTY LIVER

1. **Prioritize complete Foods:** Emphasize complete, unprocessed foods such as fruits, vegetables, whole grains, and lean meats. These meals are rich in important nutrients and fiber, promoting overall liver function.

2. **Choose Healthy Fats:** Opt for sources of healthy fats, like avocados, nuts, seeds, and olive oil. Limit saturated and Tran's fats found in fried meals, processed snacks, and fatty cuts of meat.

3. **Control Portion Sizes:** Be cautious of portion sizes to limit calorie intake. Overeating, even with nutritious meals, may lead to excess calorie intake and weight gain.

4. **Limit Added Sugars:** Reduce the consumption of meals and drinks rich in added sugars. This includes sugary beverages, candies, and processed food. High sugar consumption might lead to fat formation in the liver.

5. **Moderate Alcohol Consumption:** If ingesting alcohol, do it in moderation. Excessive alcohol consumption is a recognized risk factor for fatty liver, and moderation is vital for liver health.

6. **Stay Hydrated:** Adequate hydration is vital for general health, including liver function. Water helps remove pollutants from the body and promotes different physiological functions.

7. **Include Lean Proteins:** Choose lean protein sources such as chicken, fish, tofu, and lentils. Protein is crucial for maintaining muscle mass and promoting the regeneration of liver tissues.

8. **Prioritize Omega-3 Fatty Acids:** Include sources of omega-3 fatty acids, such as fatty fish (salmon, mackerel), flaxseeds, and walnuts. These may have anti-inflammatory properties and enhance heart health.

9. **Monitor Sodium Intake:** Keep sodium consumption in control, since excessive salt may lead to fluid retention and high blood pressure. Choose fresh, less processed foods and season dishes with herbs and spices instead of salt.

10. **Gradual Weight Management:** If overweight, strive for gradual and sustained weight reduction. Crash diets may release stored fat into the circulation, thereby aggravating fatty liver. Consult with a healthcare expert for tailored weight control assistance.

Oatmeal with Berries

Cooking Time: 10 minutes | **Prep Time:** 5 minutes | **Total Time:** 15 minutes | **Serving Size:** 1

Ingredients:
- 1/2 cup old-fashioned rolled oats
- 1 cup water or milk (dairy or plant-based)
- A pinch of salt
- 1/2 cup mixed berries (strawberries, blueberries, raspberries)
- 1 tablespoon chia seeds
- 1 tablespoon chopped nuts (almonds, walnuts, or your preference)
- 1 teaspoon honey or maple syrup (optional for sweetness)
- Fresh mint leaves for garnish (optional)

Directions:

1. **Prepare the Oats:** In a small saucepan, bring water or milk to a gentle boil. Add a pinch of salt to enhance the flavor.
2. **Add the Oats:** Stir in the old-fashioned rolled oats, reduce the heat to low, and simmer. Cook for about 5-7 minutes, stirring occasionally, until the oats are tender and have absorbed most of the liquid.
3. **Incorporate Berries:** Gently fold in the mixed berries. The heat from the oats will soften the berries and release their natural sweetness.
4. **Include Chia Seeds:** Sprinkle chia seeds over the oatmeal. Chia seeds add a boost of fiber and omega-3 fatty acids.
5. **Optional Sweetener:** If desired, drizzle honey or maple syrup over the oatmeal for added sweetness. Adjust the amount based on your taste preference.
6. **Top with Nuts:** Sprinkle chopped nuts over the oatmeal. This provides a delightful crunch and adds healthy fats.
7. **Garnish and Serve:** Once the oatmeal has reached your desired consistency, remove it from the heat. Transfer to a bowl and garnish with fresh mint leaves if you like.
8. **Enjoy Warm:** Serve the oatmeal warm and savor the wholesome combination of hearty oats and vibrant berries.

Nutritional Information (Approximate): Calories: 300 kcal, Protein: 10g, Fat: 8g, Carbohydrates: 50g, Fiber: 8g, Sugars: 12g

Greek Yogurt Parfait

Prep Time: 10 minutes | **Cooking Time:** 10 minutes | **Total Time:** 10 minutes | **Serving Size:** 1 parfait

Ingredients:

- 1 cup Greek yogurt (unsweetened)
- 1/2 cup granola (choose a low-sugar, whole-grain option)
- 1/2 cup mixed berries (strawberries, blueberries, raspberries)
- 1 tablespoon honey or maple syrup (optional)
- 1 tablespoon chopped nuts (almonds, walnuts, or your choice)

Directions:

1. **Prepare Ingredients:** Gather the Greek yogurt, granola, mixed berries, honey or maple syrup (if using), and chopped nuts.
2. **Layer the Base:** In a clear glass or bowl, spoon a layer of Greek yogurt at the bottom. Greek yogurt is high in protein and provides a creamy base for the parfait.
3. **Add Granola Layer:** Sprinkle a layer of granola over the Greek yogurt. Opt for a granola with low added sugars and whole-grain ingredients for added fiber.
4. **Berry Layer:** Add a layer of mixed berries on top of the granola. Berries are rich in antioxidants and provide a burst of natural sweetness.
5. **Repeat Layers:** Repeat the layers until you reach the top of the glass, finishing with a sprinkle of granola and a few berries.
6. **Drizzle with Honey (Optional):** If desired, drizzle a small amount of honey or maple syrup over the top for added sweetness. Adjust the amount based on your preference.
7. **Top with Chopped Nuts:** Finish the parfait by sprinkling chopped nuts over the top. Nuts add a delightful crunch and provide healthy fats.
8. **Serve Immediately:** Serve the Greek Yogurt Parfait immediately to enjoy the contrasting textures and flavors. The parfait is visually appealing with its colorful layers.
9. **Variations:** Experiment with different fruits, seeds, or flavored Greek yogurt for variety. Consider adding a dollop of nut butter for extra richness.
10. **Enjoy Mindfully:** Sit down, savor each bite, and appreciate the wholesome goodness of this nutritious and satisfying breakfast option.

Nutritional Information (per serving): Calories: 350, Protein: 20g, Fat: 15g, Carbohydrates: 40g, Fiber: 6g, Sugars: 16g

Avocado bread with Whole Grain Bread

Prep Time: 10 minutes | **Cooking Time:** 5 minutes | **Total Time:** 15 minutes | **Serving Size:** 1 parfait

Ingredient

- 1 slice whole grain bread
- 1 ripe avocado
- 1 tablespoon lemon juice
- Salt and pepper to taste
- 1/2 cup Greek yogurt
- 1 tablespoon honey
- Fresh berries for garnish (optional)
- Chia seeds for garnish (optional)

Directions:

1. **Prepare Avocado Spread:** Mash the ripe avocado in a bowl then Add lemon juice, salt, and pepper to taste, Mix well to create a smooth avocado spread.

2. **Toast Whole Grain Bread:** Toast the whole grain bread until it reaches your desired level of crispiness.

3. **Assemble Parfait:** Cut the toasted bread into bite-sized cubes In a glass or parfait dish, layer half of the avocado spread at the bottom then Add a layer of whole grain bread cubes on top of the avocado. Spoon half of the Greek yogurt over the bread layer and Drizzle with half of the honey.

4. **Repeat Layers:** Repeat the layers using the remaining avocado spread, bread cubes, Greek yogurt, and honey.

5. **Garnish:** Top the parfait with fresh berries for a burst of color and added antioxidants and Sprinkle chia seeds for an extra boost of fiber and nutrients.

6. **Serve:** Serve immediately, allowing the flavors to meld together.

Nutritional Information per Serving: Calories: 350 kcal, **Protein:** 10g, **Fat:** 22g, **Carbohydrates:** 32g, **Fiber:** 8g

Vegetable Omelette

Prep Time: 10 minutes | **Cooking Time:** 10 minutes | **Total Time:** 20 minutes | **Servings:** 1

Ingredients:

- 2 large eggs
- 1/4 cup diced bell peppers (red, green, or yellow)
- 1/4 cup diced tomatoes
- 1/4 cup chopped spinach
- 1/4 cup diced onions
- 1 tablespoon olive oil
- Salt and pepper to taste
- 1/2 teaspoon dried herbs (such as oregano or thyme)

Directions:

1. **Prep the Vegetables:** Dice bell peppers, tomatoes, and onions and Chop spinach.

2. **Sauté Vegetables:** Heat olive oil in a non-stick skillet over medium heat. Add diced onions and cook until translucent, Add bell peppers and tomatoes, sauté until softened and add chopped spinach and cook until wilted.

3. **Beat Eggs:** In a bowl, beat the eggs until well mixed then Season with salt, pepper, and dried herbs.

4. **Combine and Cook:** Pour the beaten eggs over the sautéed vegetables in the skillet and allow the eggs to set around the edges, gently lifting them with a spatula to let the uncooked eggs flow underneath, once the omelette is mostly set but still slightly runny on top, fold it in half.

5. **Finish Cooking:** Continue cooking for another minute or until the eggs are fully set but still moist.

6. **Serve:** Slide the omelette onto a plate and Garnish with additional herbs if desired.

Nutritional Information per serving: Serving Size: 1 omelette, Calories: Approximately 250 kcal, Protein: 14g, Fat: 18g, Carbohydrates: 8g, Fiber: 2g

Smoothie Bowl

Prep Time: 10 minutes | **Cooking Time:** 10 minutes | **Total Time:** 10 minutes | **Serving Size:** 1

Ingredients:

- 1 cup mixed berries (strawberries, blueberries, raspberries)
- 1 small ripe banana
- 1/2 cup spinach leaves, washed
- 1/4 cup chia seeds
- 1 tablespoon flaxseeds
- 1 tablespoon almond butter
- 1/2 cup unsweetened almond milk
- 1/2 cup plain Greek yogurt
- 1 teaspoon honey (optional, for sweetness)
- Ice cubes (optional)

Directions:

1. **Gather Ingredients:** Collect all the ingredients in one place.

2. **Prepare Fruits:** Wash the berries thoroughly and peel the banana.

3. **Blend Fruits and Vegetables:** In a blender, combine the mixed berries, banana, spinach leaves, chia seeds, flaxseeds, almond butter, almond milk, and Greek yogurt.

4. **Blend until Smooth:** Blend the ingredients until you achieve a smooth and creamy consistency. If the mixture is too thick, you can add more almond milk.

5. **Taste and Sweeten:** Taste the smoothie and add honey if desired, depending on your sweetness preference.

6. **Prepare Toppings:** Pour the smoothie into a bowl and add your favorite toppings. Consider sliced strawberries, banana slices, a sprinkle of chia seeds, or a dollop of Greek yogurt.

7. **Serve Immediately:** Enjoy the smoothie bowl immediately to preserve its freshness.

Nutritional Information (approximate): Calories: 300 kcal, Total Fat: 10g, Saturated Fat: 2g, Cholesterol: 0mg, Sodium: 20mg, Total Carbohydrates: 45g, Dietary Fiber: 10g, Sugars: 20g, Protein: 12g

Quinoa Breakfast Bowl

Prep Time: 10 minutes | **Cooking Time:** 15 minutes | **Total Time:** 25 minutes | **Serving Size:** 2

Ingredients:

- 1 cup quinoa, rinsed
- 2 cups water
- 1 tablespoon olive oil
- 1 medium onion, diced
- 1 bell pepper, diced
- 1 zucchini, diced
- 2 cloves garlic, minced
- 1 teaspoon turmeric powder
- Salt and pepper to taste
- 2 cups spinach, chopped
- 4 eggs
- 1 avocado, sliced (optional)
- Fresh herbs for garnish (parsley, cilantro)

Directions:

1. **Cook Quinoa:** In a medium saucepan, combine rinsed quinoa and water. Bring to a boil, then reduce heat to low, cover, and simmer for 15 minutes or until water is absorbed. Fluff with a fork.

2. **Prepare Vegetables:** In a large skillet, heat olive oil over medium heat. Add diced onion, bell pepper, zucchini, and minced garlic. Sauté until vegetables are tender, about 5-7 minutes.

3. **Season with Turmeric:** Stir in turmeric powder, salt, and pepper. Cook for an additional 2 minutes, allowing the flavors to meld.

4. **Add Spinach:** Add chopped spinach to the skillet and cook until wilted. Remove the skillet from heat.

5. **Cook Eggs:** In a separate non-stick pan, cook eggs to your liking (poached or fried).

6. **Assemble Bowls:** Divide the cooked quinoa among two bowls. Top with the sautéed vegetable mixture and place the cooked eggs on top.

7. **Garnish and Serve:** Garnish with fresh herbs and avocado slices if desired. Serve the Quinoa Breakfast Bowls warm.

Nutritional Information (per serving): Calories: 400, Protein: 18g, Carbohydrates: 45g, Fat: 18g, Fiber: 8g

Cottage Cheese Bowl

Prep Time: 10 minutes | **Cooking Time:** 10 minutes | **Total Time:** 10 minutes | **Serving Size:** 1

Ingredients:

- 1 cup low-fat cottage cheese
- 1/2 cup fresh blueberries
- 1/2 cup sliced strawberries
- 1 tablespoon chia seeds
- 1 tablespoon flaxseeds
- 1 tablespoon honey (optional for sweetness)
- 1/4 cup chopped walnuts
- 1 teaspoon cinnamon
- Fresh mint leaves for garnish (optional)

Directions:

1. In a mixing bowl, combine the low-fat cottage cheese, chia seeds, flaxseeds, and cinnamon. Mix well to ensure an even distribution of ingredients.

2. Add fresh blueberries and sliced strawberries to the bowl. These berries are rich in antioxidants and provide a burst of flavor.

3. If you prefer a touch of sweetness, drizzle honey over the cottage cheese mixture. Adjust the amount based on your taste preferences.

4. Sprinkle chopped walnuts over the top. Walnuts are a great source of healthy fats and add a delightful crunch to the dish.

5. Gently fold all the ingredients together, ensuring the cottage cheese is well-coated with the berries, seeds, and nuts.

6. Let the mixture sit for a couple of minutes to allow the flavors to meld. This also gives the chia seeds time to absorb some liquid and achieve a pudding-like consistency.

7. Garnish with fresh mint leaves for a burst of freshness (optional).

8. Your Fatty Liver-Friendly Cottage Cheese Bowl is ready to be served! Enjoy this nutritious and delicious breakfast that is gentle on the liver while providing essential nutrients.

Nutritional Information (per serving): Calories: ~300, Protein: ~25g, Carbohydrates: ~25g, Healthy Fats: ~12g, Fiber: ~5g

Turmeric Infused Golden Milk Smoothie

Prep Time: 10 minutes | **Cooking Time**: 10 minutes | **Total Time:** 10 minutes | **Serving Size:** 2 servings

Ingredients:
- 1 ripe banana, frozen
- 1/2 cup plain Greek yogurt
- 1 cup unsweetened almond milk
- 1 tablespoon chia seeds
- 1 tablespoon ground flaxseed
- 1 teaspoon turmeric powder
- 1/2 teaspoon cinnamon
- 1/4 teaspoon ginger powder
- 1/4 teaspoon black pepper (enhances turmeric absorption)
- 1 tablespoon honey or maple syrup (optional, for sweetness)
- Ice cubes (optional)

Directions:

1. **Prepare Ingredients:** Peel and freeze a ripe banana the night before and Measure out chia seeds, ground flaxseed, turmeric powder, cinnamon, ginger powder, and set aside.

2. **Blend Smoothie:** In a blender, combine the frozen banana, Greek yogurt, almond milk, chia seeds, ground flaxseed, turmeric powder, cinnamon, ginger powder, and black pepper, Blend until smooth and creamy. Add ice cubes if you prefer a colder consistency.

3. **Adjust Sweetness:** Taste the smoothie and add honey or maple syrup if desired. Blend again to combine.

4. **Serve:** Pour the golden milk smoothie into glasses.

5. **Garnish (Optional):** Garnish with a sprinkle of turmeric or a cinnamon stick for presentation.

6. **Enjoy:** Sip and savor the Turmeric Infused Golden Milk Smoothie, rich in anti-inflammatory properties and beneficial for fatty liver health.

Nutritional Information (per serving): Calories: 180, Total Fat: 8g, Saturated Fat: 4g, Cholesterol: 20mg, Sodium: 80mg, Total Carbohydrates: 25g, Dietary Fiber: 5g, Sugars: 15g, Protein: 7g, Vitamin D: 10%, Calcium: 20%, Iron: 15%, Potassium: 10%

Grilled Salmon Salad

Prep Time: 10 minutes | **Cook Time**: 15 minutes | **Total Time**: 25 minutes | **Servings**: 2

Ingredients:

- 2 (6-ounce) salmon fillets
- 1 tablespoon olive oil
- 1/2 teaspoon dried oregano
- 1/4 teaspoon garlic powder
- Salt and pepper to taste
- 2 cups mixed greens
- 1/2 cup cherry tomatoes, halved
- 1/4 cup cucumber, diced
- 1/4 cup red onion, thinly sliced
- 1/4 cup crumbled feta cheese (optional)
- 2 tablespoons olive oil and lemon juice vinaigrette

Directions:

1. Preheat grill to medium-high heat.
2. In a small bowl, combine olive oil, oregano, garlic powder, salt, and pepper. Rub the mixture onto the salmon fillets.
3. Place the salmon fillets on the preheated grill and cook for 5-7 minutes per side, or until cooked through.
4. While the salmon is cooking, prepare the salad by combining the mixed greens, tomatoes, cucumber, and red onion in a large bowl.
5. Once the salmon is cooked, flake it into bite-sized pieces and add it to the salad bowl.
6. Drizzle the salad with the olive oil and lemon juice vinaigrette and toss to coat.
7. Serve immediately, topped with crumbled feta cheese (optional).

Nutritional Information: Calories: 450, Fat: 25g, Saturated Fat: 5g, Carbohydrates: 15g, Fiber: 3g, Protein: 35g, Sodium: 300mg

Quinoa and Vegetable Stir-Fry

Cooking Time: 15 minutes | **Prep Time**: 10 minutes | **Total Time**: 25 minutes | **Servings**: 2

Ingredients:

- 1 cup quinoa, rinsed
- 1 1/2 cups vegetable broth
- 1 tablespoon olive oil
- 1 onion, chopped
- 2 cloves garlic, minced
- 1 bell pepper, chopped
- 1 cup broccoli florets
- 1/2 cup cherry tomatoes
- 1/4 cup chopped fresh cilantro
- 1/4 teaspoon sea salt
- 1/4 teaspoon black pepper
- 1/2 lemon, juiced (optional)

Directions:

1. In a medium saucepan, combine the quinoa and vegetable broth. Bring to a boil, then reduce heat, cover, and simmer for 15 minutes, or until the quinoa is cooked through and fluffy.
2. Meanwhile, heat the olive oil in a large skillet or wok over medium heat. Add the onion and garlic and cook, stirring occasionally, until softened, about 5 minutes.
3. Add the bell pepper, broccoli, and tomatoes to the skillet and cook, stirring occasionally, for 5-7 minutes, or until the vegetables are tender-crisp.
4. Stir in the cooked quinoa, cilantro, salt, and pepper. Cook for an additional minute or two, until everything is heated through.
5. Serve immediately, with a squeeze of lemon juice, if desired.

Nutritional Information per Serving: Calories: 350, Fat: 8g, Saturated Fat: 2g, Cholesterol: 0mg, Carbohydrates: 45g, Fiber: 6g, Protein: 15g

Turkey and Avocado Wrap

Prep time: 10 minutes | **Cooking time**: 5 minutes | **Total time**: 15 minutes | **Serving size**: 1 wrap

Ingredients:

- 1 whole-wheat tortilla
- 4 ounces sliced cooked turkey breast
- 1/4 avocado, sliced
- 1 tomato, sliced
- 1/4 cup shredded romaine lettuce
- 1 tablespoon hummus
- 1 teaspoon Dijon mustard
- Salt and pepper to taste

Directions:

1. Spread the hummus and Dijon mustard over the tortilla.

2. Layer the turkey, avocado, tomato, and lettuce on top of the hummus mixture.

3. Season with salt and pepper to taste.

4. Roll up the tortilla tightly and enjoy!

Nutritional information: Calories: 380, Fat: 14g, Saturated fat: 3g, Carbohydrates: 24g, Fiber: 7g, Protein: 32g

Vegetable and Lentil Soup

Prep time: 10 minutes | **Cook time**: 30 minutes | **Total time**: 40 minutes | **Servings**: 4

Ingredients:

- 1 tablespoon olive oil
- 1 onion, chopped
- 2 carrots, chopped
- 2 celery stalks, chopped
- 2 cloves garlic, minced
- 1 teaspoon ground cumin
- 1/2 teaspoon smoked paprika
- 1/4 teaspoon cayenne pepper (optional)
- 4 cups vegetable broth
- 1 cup green lentils, rinsed
- 1 (14.5-ounce) can diced tomatoes, undrained
- 1 (15-ounce) can black beans, rinsed and drained
- 1 cup frozen corn
- 1/2 cup chopped fresh cilantro
- Salt and pepper to taste

Directions:

1. Heat olive oil in a large pot over medium heat. Add onion, carrots, and celery and cook until softened, about 5 minutes.

2. Add garlic, cumin, paprika, and cayenne pepper (if using) and cook for 1 minute more.

3. Stir in vegetable broth, lentils, tomatoes, black beans, and corn. Bring to a boil, then reduce heat and simmer for 20 minutes, or until lentils are tender.

4. Stir in cilantro and season with salt and pepper to taste.

5. Serve hot.

Nutritional information per serving: Calories: 320, Fat: 7g, Saturated fat: 1g, Cholesterol: 0mg, Sodium: 350mg, Carbohydrates: 48g, Fiber: 13g, Sugar: 8g, Protein: 18g

Baked Chicken Breast with Sweet Potato

Cooking Time: 35 minutes | **Prep Time**: 10 minutes | **Total Time**: 45 minutes | **Serving Size**: 2

Ingredients:

- 2 boneless, skinless chicken breasts
- 1 medium sweet potato, peeled and diced
- 1 tablespoon olive oil
- 1/2 teaspoon dried thyme
- 1/4 teaspoon garlic powder
- 1/4 teaspoon salt
- 1/4 teaspoon black pepper
- 1/4 cup water

Directions:

1. Preheat oven to 400 degrees F (200 degrees C). Line a baking sheet with parchment paper.

2. In a small bowl, combine olive oil, thyme, garlic powder, salt, and pepper.

3. Rub the chicken breasts with the spice mixture.

4. Place the chicken breasts on the prepared baking sheet.

5. Around the chicken, scatter the diced sweet potato.

6. Pour the water into the bottom of the baking sheet.

7. Bake for 35 minutes, or until the chicken is cooked through and the sweet potato is tender.

8. Serve immediately.

Nutritional Information: Calories: 400, Protein: 40g, Fat: 10g, Carbohydrates: 30g, Fiber: 5g

Quinoa and Black Bean Salad

Prep time: 10 minutes | **Cooking time**: 20 minutes | **Total time**: 30 minutes | **Servings**: 2

Ingredients:

- 1 cup quinoa, rinsed
- 1 1/2 cups water or vegetable broth
- 1/2 cup diced red onion
- 1/2 cup chopped red bell pepper
- 1 (15-ounce) can black beans, rinsed and drained
- 1/4 cup chopped fresh cilantro
- 2 tablespoons olive oil
- 2 tablespoons lime juice
- 1 tablespoon apple cider vinegar
- 1 teaspoon ground cumin
- 1/2 teaspoon chili powder
- 1/4 teaspoon salt
- 1/4 teaspoon black pepper

Directions:

1. In a medium saucepan, combine the quinoa and water or broth. Bring to a boil, then reduce heat, cover, and simmer for 15 minutes, or until the quinoa is cooked through and fluffy.

2. While the quinoa is cooking, in a large bowl, combine the red onion, bell pepper, black beans, and cilantro.

3. In a small bowl, whisk together the olive oil, lime juice, apple cider vinegar, cumin, chili powder, salt, and black pepper.

4. Once the quinoa is cooked, fluff it with a fork and add it to the bowl with the other ingredients.

5. Pour the dressing over the salad and toss to coat evenly.

6. Serve immediately or refrigerate for up to 3 days.

Nutritional information Per serving: 350 calories, 14 grams of fat, 38 grams of carbohydrates, 17 grams of protein, and 8 grams of fiber. It is also a good source of iron, magnesium, and potassium.

Grilled Shrimp and Vegetable Skewers

Prep Time: 15 minutes | **Cook Time**: 10 minutes | **Total Time**: 25 minutes | **Serving Size**: 2 skewers

Ingredients:

- 12 large shrimp, peeled and deveined
- 1 bell pepper, cut into chunks
- 1 red onion, cut into chunks
- 1 zucchini, cut into chunks
- 1 tablespoon olive oil
- 1/2 teaspoon dried oregano
- 1/4 teaspoon garlic powder
- Salt and pepper to taste
- Wooden skewers

Directions:

1. Preheat your grill to medium-high heat.

2. In a bowl, toss the shrimp, bell pepper, onion, and zucchini with olive oil, oregano, garlic powder, salt, and pepper.

3. Thread the shrimp and vegetables onto skewers, alternating between shrimp and vegetables.

4. Grill the skewers for 5-7 minutes per side, or until the shrimp are cooked through and the vegetables are tender.

5. Serve immediately with your favorite dipping sauce, such as a low-fat yogurt-based sauce or a simple vinaigrette.

Nutritional Information: Calories: 300, Fat: 8g, Carbohydrates: 15g, Fiber: 3g, Protein: 25g

Spinach and Feta Stuffed Chicken Breast

Prep Time: 15 minutes | **Cook Time**: 30 minutes | **Total Time**: 45 minutes | **Servings**: 4

Ingredients:

- 4 boneless, skinless chicken breasts
- 1 tablespoon olive oil
- 1/2 onion, diced
- 2 cloves garlic, minced
- 5 ounces baby spinach
- 1/2 cup crumbled feta cheese
- 1/4 cup chopped fresh parsley
- 1/4 teaspoon dried oregano
- 1/4 teaspoon salt
- 1/4 teaspoon black pepper

Directions:

1. Preheat oven to 375 degrees F (190 degrees C).

2. In a large skillet, heat olive oil over medium heat. Add onion and cook until softened, about 5 minutes. Add garlic and cook for an additional minute.

3. Stir in spinach and cook until wilted, about 2 minutes.

4. Remove from heat and stir in feta cheese, parsley, oregano, salt, and pepper.

5. Using a sharp knife, carefully make a pocket in each chicken breast. Be sure not to cut all the way through.

6. Stuff each pocket with the spinach and feta mixture.

7. Place chicken breasts in a baking dish and bake for 30 minutes, or until cooked through.

8. Serve immediately.

Nutritional Information: Calories: 300, Fat: 8g, Saturated Fat: 2g, Cholesterol: 70mg, Sodium: 250mg, Carbohydrates: 5g, Fiber: 2g, Sugar: 1g, Protein: 40g

Mushroom and Spinach Omelette

Prep time: 5 minutes | **Cooking time**: 10 minutes | **Total time**: 15 minutes | **Serving size**: 1

Ingredients:

- 2 eggs
- 1 tablespoon olive oil
- 1/2 cup chopped mushrooms
- 1/2 cup chopped spinach
- 1/4 cup chopped onion
- 1/4 cup chopped tomato
- 1/4 teaspoon dried oregano
- Salt and pepper to taste

Directions:

1. Heat olive oil in a non-stick skillet over medium heat. Add onion and cook until softened, about 3 minutes.

2. Add mushrooms and cook until browned, about 5 minutes.

3. Add spinach and cook until wilted, about 1 minute.

4. Add oregano, salt, and pepper to taste.

5. In a separate bowl, whisk together eggs.

6. Pour egg mixture into the skillet and cook until the bottom is set, about 2 minutes.

7. Use a spatula to fold the omelette in half.

8. Cook for an additional minute or two, or until the eggs are cooked through.

9. Serve immediately.

Nutritional information: Calories: 300, Protein: 20g, Fat: 20g, Carbohydrates: 5g

Cauliflower Rice Bowl with Tofu

Prep time: 15 minutes | **Cook time**: 20 minutes | **Total time**: 35 minutes | **Serving size**: 2

Ingredients:

- 1 head of cauliflower, riced
- 1 block of firm tofu, cubed
- 1 tablespoon olive oil
- 1/2 teaspoon ground ginger
- 1/4 teaspoon garlic powder
- 1/4 teaspoon red pepper flakes (optional)
- 1/4 cup low-sodium soy sauce
- 1 tablespoon rice vinegar
- 1 tablespoon honey
- 1 tablespoon sesame oil
- 1/2 cup chopped vegetables, such as carrots, bell peppers, broccoli
- 1/4 cup chopped green onions
- 1 tablespoon sesame seeds

Directions:

1. Heat olive oil in a large skillet over medium heat. Add tofu and cook until golden brown on all sides, about 5 minutes per side.

2. Add ginger, garlic powder, and red pepper flakes (if using) to the skillet and cook for 30 seconds, until fragrant.

3. Add soy sauce, rice vinegar, honey, and sesame oil to the skillet and bring to a simmer. Cook for 5 minutes, until sauce thickens slightly.

4. Add cauliflower rice and chopped vegetables to the skillet and cook until cauliflower rice is heated through, about 5 minutes.

5. Serve immediately topped with green onions and sesame seeds.

Nutritional information per serving: Calories: 340, Fat: 10g, Carbohydrates: 25g, Fiber: 5g, Protein: 20g

Guacamole with Veggie Sticks

Prep Time: 15 minutes | **Cooking Time:** 0 minutes | **Total Time:** 15 minutes | **Serving Size:** 4

Ingredients:

- 3 ripe avocados
- 1 small red onion, finely diced
- 2 tomatoes, diced
- 1 clove garlic, minced
- 1 lime, juiced
- 1/4 cup fresh cilantro, chopped
- Salt and pepper to taste

Veggie Sticks:
- Carrot sticks
- Cucumber slices
- Bell pepper strips

Directions:

1. **Prepare Vegetables:** Wash and cut the carrots, cucumber, and bell peppers into sticks and slices for dipping.

2. **Guacamole Base:** Cut the avocados in half, remove the pits, and scoop the flesh into a bowl Mash the avocados using a fork or potato masher until smooth.

3. **Mixing:** Add the diced red onion, tomatoes, minced garlic, and chopped cilantro to the mashed avocados Squeeze the juice of one lime into the mixture Season with salt and pepper to taste.

4. **Combine Thoroughly:** Gently fold all the ingredients together until well combined. Be careful not to over-mix to maintain a chunky texture.

5. **Adjust Seasoning:** Taste the guacamole and adjust the lime, salt, and pepper to suit your preference.

6. **Serve:** Place the guacamole in a serving bowl and surround it with the prepared veggie sticks.

7. **Enjoy:** Dip the veggie sticks into the guacamole and savor the creamy, flavorful snack.

Nutritional Information (per serving): Calories: Approximately 200 kcal, **Fat:** 15g, **Carbohydrates:** 17g, **Protein:** 3g, **Fiber:** 9g

Hummus with Whole Grain Crackers

Prep Time: 15 minutes | **Cooking Time:** 0 minutes | **Total Time:** 15 minutes | **Serving Size:** 6

Ingredients:

- 1 can (15 oz) chickpeas, drained and rinsed
- 1/4 cup extra virgin olive oil
- 1/4 cup water
- 1/3 cup tahini
- 2 cloves garlic, minced
- 1 teaspoon ground cumin
- 1/2 teaspoon salt (or to taste)
- 1/4 teaspoon paprika (for garnish)
- Whole grain crackers (choose low-sodium varieties)

Directions:

1. **Prepare Chickpeas:** Rinse and drain the canned chickpeas.

2. **Blend Ingredients:** In a food processor, combine chickpeas, olive oil, water, tahini, minced garlic, cumin, and salt. Blend until smooth, scraping down the sides as needed.

3. **Adjust Consistency:** If the hummus is too thick, add more water, a tablespoon at a time, until you reach the desired consistency.

4. **Serve:** Transfer the hummus to a serving bowl. Drizzle with a bit of extra virgin olive oil and sprinkle paprika for garnish.

5. **Pair with Whole Grain Crackers:** Serve the hummus with a selection of whole grain crackers. Choose crackers with minimal added salt to keep the snack liver-friendly.

6. **Enjoy:** Serve immediately and enjoy your tasty, fatty liver-friendly hummus with whole grain crackers.

Nutritional Information (per serving): Calories: 180, Total Fat: 14g, Saturated Fat: 2g, Cholesterol: 0mg, Sodium: 200mg, Carbohydrates: 10g, Dietary Fiber: 3g, Sugars: 1g, Protein: 4g

Greek Yogurt with Berries

Prep Time: 10 minutes | **Cook Time:** 0 minutes | **Total Time:** 10 minutes | **Serving Size:** 2

Ingredients:

- 1 cup plain Greek yogurt (preferably low-fat)
- 1/2 cup mixed berries (blueberries, raspberries, strawberries)
- 1 tablespoon chia seeds
- 1 tablespoon honey (optional, for sweetness)
- 1/4 teaspoon vanilla extract
- 1 tablespoon chopped nuts (almonds or walnuts)
- Fresh mint leaves for garnish (optional)

Directions:

1. **Prepare the Berries:** Rinse the berries thoroughly and pat them dry with a paper towel. If using strawberries, hull and slice them.

2. **Mix the Yogurt:** In a mixing bowl, combine the Greek yogurt, chia seeds, vanilla extract, and honey (if using). Stir the mixture until well combined.

3. **Assemble the Dish:** In serving bowls or glasses, layer the Greek yogurt mixture and berries. Add a sprinkle of chopped nuts on top.

4. **Garnish and Serve:** Garnish with fresh mint leaves for a burst of freshness. Drizzle a bit more honey on top if desired.

5. **Enjoy:** Serve immediately and enjoy this delicious and nutritious snack.

Nutritional Information (per serving): Calories: ~150, Protein: ~15g, Carbohydrates: ~15g, Fat: ~5g, Fiber: ~4g

Roasted Chickpeas

Prep Time: 10 minutes | **Cook Time:** 30 minutes | **Total Time:** 40 minutes | **Serving Size:** 4

Ingredients:

- 2 cans (15 oz each) chickpeas, drained and rinsed
- 2 tablespoons olive oil
- 1 teaspoon dried oregano
- 1 teaspoon dried thyme
- 1 teaspoon garlic powder
- 1 teaspoon onion powder
- 1/2 teaspoon paprika
- Salt and pepper to taste

Directions:

1. **Preheat the Oven:** Preheat your oven to 400°F (200°C).

2. **Prepare Chickpeas:** Pat dry the rinsed chickpeas using a kitchen towel. Remove any loose skins.

3. **Seasoning:** In a large bowl, toss chickpeas with olive oil, oregano, thyme, garlic powder, onion powder, paprika, salt, and pepper. Ensure an even coating.

4. **Spread on Baking Sheet:** Spread the seasoned chickpeas in a single layer on a baking sheet. This ensures even roasting.

5. **Roasting:** Roast the chickpeas in the preheated oven for about 30 minutes or until they are golden brown and crunchy. Shake the pan or stir the chickpeas halfway through the cooking time for even crispiness.

6. **Cooling:** Allow the roasted chickpeas to cool for a few minutes before serving.

7. **Serve:** Serve as a delightful snack or appetizer. They can be enjoyed warm or at room temperature.

Nutritional Information (per serving): Calories: 220, Total Fat: 8g, Saturated Fat: 1g, Trans Fat: 0g, Cholesterol: 0mg, Sodium: 300mg, Total Carbohydrates: 30g, Dietary Fiber: 7g, Sugars: 5g, Protein: 8g

Caprese Skewers

Prep Time: 15 minutes | **Cooking Time:** 0 minutes | **Total Time:** 15 minutes | **Serving Size:** 4

Ingredients:

- Cherry tomatoes
- Fresh mozzarella balls
- Fresh basil leaves
- Extra virgin olive oil
- Balsamic vinegar
- Salt and pepper to taste

Directions:

1. **Prepare Ingredients:** Wash cherry tomatoes and basil leaves. Drain fresh mozzarella balls if stored in liquid.

2. **Assemble Skewers:** On small skewers or toothpicks, thread one cherry tomato, one mozzarella ball, and one basil leaf. Repeat until the skewer is filled, leaving a bit of space at each end.

3. **Arrange Skewers:** Place the assembled skewers on a serving platter or dish.

4. **Seasoning:** Drizzle extra virgin olive oil and balsamic vinegar over the skewers. Sprinkle with a pinch of salt and pepper to taste.

5. **Chill:** Refrigerate the skewers for at least 30 minutes before serving. This enhances the flavors and makes them refreshing.

6. **Serve:** Arrange the Caprese Skewers on a serving dish. Garnish with additional fresh basil if desired.

7. **Enjoy:** These Caprese Skewers make a delightful and liver-friendly snack or appetizer. Serve them at parties, gatherings, or as a healthy snack option.

Nutritional Information (per serving): Calories: 150, Total Fat: 10g, Saturated Fat: 5g, Cholesterol: 25mg, Sodium: 200mg, Total Carbohydrates: 5g, Dietary Fiber: 1g, Sugars: 2g, Protein: 8g

Veggie Sushi Rolls

Prep Time: 15-20 minutes | **Cooking Time**: 20-25 minutes | **Total Time**: 40 minutes | **Serving Size**: 6 Rolls

Ingredients:
- 1 cup sushi rice
- 2 tablespoons rice vinegar
- 1 tablespoon sugar
- 1/2 teaspoon salt
- Nori seaweed sheets
- Carrots, julienned
- Cucumber, julienned
- Avocado, sliced
- Radishes, thinly sliced
- Sesame seeds
- Low-sodium soy sauce for dipping
- Pickled ginger and wasabi (optional)

Directions:

1. **Preparation:** Rinse the sushi rice under cold water until the water runs clear. Cook the rice according to package instructions. While still hot, mix in rice vinegar, sugar, and salt. Allow it to cool.

2. **Rolling Station:** Place a bamboo sushi rolling mat on a flat surface. Lay a sheet of plastic wrap on the mat, followed by a sheet of nori, shiny side down.

3. **Rice and Filling:** Wet your hands to prevent the rice from sticking, then spread a thin layer of rice over the nori, leaving about an inch at the top. Arrange a small amount of each veggie filling horizontally across the center of the rice.

4. **Rolling:** Lift the edge of the mat closest to you and begin rolling it away from you, using gentle pressure. Seal the edge of the nori with a little water to secure the roll.

5. **Cutting:** Use a sharp, wet knife to cut the roll into bite-sized pieces.

6. **Presentation:** Arrange the sushi rolls on a plate, sprinkle with sesame seeds, and garnish with additional sliced veggies.

Nut combination

Cooking Time: 15-20 minutes | **Prep Time:** 10 minutes | **Total Time:** 30 minutes | **Serving Size:** 2

Ingredients:

- 1 cup raw almonds
- 1 cup walnuts
- 1/2 cup pumpkin seeds
- 1/2 cup sunflower seeds
- 1 tablespoon olive oil
- 1 teaspoon sea salt (optional)
- 1/2 teaspoon turmeric powder
- 1/2 teaspoon cumin powder
- 1/2 teaspoon paprika

Directions:

1. **Preheat the Oven:** Preheat your oven to 325°F (163°C).

2. **Prepare the Nuts:** In a large mixing bowl, combine almonds, walnuts, pumpkin seeds, and sunflower seeds.

3. **Season the Nuts:** Drizzle olive oil over the nuts and toss them to coat evenly. Sprinkle turmeric powder, cumin powder, and paprika. Add sea salt if desired. Mix well to ensure the nuts are evenly coated with the seasoning.

4. **Spread on Baking Sheet:** Spread the seasoned nuts in a single layer on a baking sheet lined with parchment paper.

5. **Bake:** Bake in the preheated oven for 15-20 minutes or until the nuts are golden brown, stirring once halfway through.

6. **Cooling:** Allow the nuts to cool completely on the baking sheet. They will crisp up as they cool.

7. **Store:** Once cooled, transfer the nut combination to an airtight container for storage.

Nutritional Information: Calories: Approximately 200 kcal, Protein: 8g, Fat: 18g, Carbohydrates: 5g, Fiber: 3g

Edamame with Sea Salt

Prep Time: 5 minutes | **Cook Time:** 5 minutes | **Total Time:** 10 minutes | **Serving Size:** 1 cup

Ingredients:

- 2 cups frozen edamame (in pods)
- 1 tablespoon sea salt

Directions:

1. **Preparation:** Thaw the frozen edamame if necessary. Set a pot of water to boil.

2. **Cooking Time:** Boil the edamame for 3-5 minutes or until they are tender.

3. **Drain and Cool:** Drain the edamame in a colander and let them cool for a few minutes.

4. **Seasoning:** Sprinkle the boiled edamame with sea salt evenly.

5. **Toss and Serve:** Toss the edamame gently to coat them evenly with the sea salt. Serve them in a bowl or on a plate.

Nutritional Information: Calories: Approximately 120 kcalProtein: 11gCarbohydrates: 9gFiber: 5gFat: 5gSodium: 1750mg

Stuffed Bell Peppers

Prep Time: 20 minutes | **Cook Time:** 40 minutes | **Total Time:** 1 hour | **Serving Size:** 4

Ingredients
- 4 large bell peppers (choose colorful ones)
- 1 lb. lean ground turkey or chicken
- 1 cup quinoa (rinsed)
- 1 cup black beans (canned, drained, and rinsed)
- 1 cup corn kernels (fresh or frozen)
- 1 cup diced tomatoes
- 1 cup low-fat shredded cheese
- 1 teaspoon olive oil
- 1 teaspoon cumin
- 1 teaspoon garlic powder
- 1 teaspoon paprika
- Salt and pepper to taste
- Fresh cilantro for garnish (optional)

Directions:
1. **Preheat the Oven:** Preheat your oven to 375°F (190°C).
2. **Prepare Bell Peppers:** Cut the tops off the bell peppers, removing seeds and membranes. Lightly brush the outsides with olive oil.
3. **Cook Quinoa:** Rinse quinoa under cold water. In a saucepan, combine 1 cup quinoa with 2 cups of water. Bring to a boil, then reduce heat, cover, and simmer for 15-20 minutes or until quinoa is cooked. Set aside.
4. **Cook Turkey/Chicken:** In a skillet over medium heat, cook the ground turkey or chicken until browned. Season with cumin, garlic powder, paprika, salt, and pepper.
5. **Mix Ingredients:** In a large bowl, combine the cooked quinoa, browned meat, black beans, corn, diced tomatoes, and half of the shredded cheese. Mix well.
6. **Stuff Bell Peppers:** Stuff each bell pepper with the mixture, pressing it down gently. Top each pepper with the remaining shredded cheese.
7. **Bake:** Place the stuffed peppers in a baking dish. Bake in the preheated oven for 25-30 minutes or until the peppers are tender.
8. **Garnish and Serve:** Once out of the oven, garnish with fresh cilantro if desired. Allow them to cool for a few minutes before serving.

Nutritional Information per serving: Calories: ~400, Protein: ~25g, Carbohydrates: ~45g, Fat: ~15g, Fiber: ~8g

Cucumber Roll-Ups with Turkey and Cheese

Prep Time: 15 minutes | **Cook Time:** 0 minutes | **Total Time:** 15 minutes | **Servings:** 4

Ingredients

- 1 large cucumber
- 8 slices of lean turkey
- 4 slices of low-fat cheese (such as Swiss or mozzarella)
- 1/4 cup low-fat cream cheese
- 1 tablespoon Dijon mustard
- Salt and pepper to taste
- Fresh dill or parsley for garnish (optional)

Directions:

1. **Prepare the Cucumber:** Wash and peel the cucumber. Using a mandolin or a vegetable peeler, slice the cucumber lengthwise into thin strips. Pat them dry with a paper towel to remove excess moisture.

2. **Make the Cream Cheese Spread:** In a small bowl, combine the low-fat cream cheese and Dijon mustard. Mix well until smooth. Season with salt and pepper to taste.

3. **Assemble the Roll-Ups:** Lay out the cucumber slices on a clean surface. Spread a thin layer of the cream cheese mixture onto each slice. Place a slice of turkey on top of the cream cheese, and then add a slice of low-fat cheese.

4. **Roll Them Up:** Carefully roll each cucumber slice with the turkey and cheese into a tight spiral. Secure with toothpicks if needed.

5. **Chill and Slice:** Place the rolled-up cucumber snacks in the refrigerator for about 10 minutes to allow them to firm up. Once chilled, remove and slice each roll into bite-sized pieces.

6. **Garnish and Serve:** Garnish with fresh dill or parsley if desired. Arrange the roll-ups on a serving platter and serve immediately.

Nutritional Information per serving: Calories: ~120, Protein: ~15g, Carbohydrates: ~5g, Fat: ~5g, Fiber: ~1g

Baked Apples with Cinnamon and Walnuts

Prep Time: 15 minutes | **Cook Time:** 30 minutes | **Total Time:** 45 minutes | **Serving Size:** 4 servings

Ingredients:
- 4 large apples (such as Granny Smith or Honey crisp)
- 1/2 cup chopped walnuts
- 2 tablespoons honey or maple syrup
- 2 tablespoons melted coconut oil
- 1 teaspoon ground cinnamon
- 1/4 teaspoon ground nutmeg
- Pinch of salt

Directions:

1. **Preheat the Oven:** Preheat your oven to 375°F (190°C).

2. **Prepare the Apples:** Wash and core the apples, removing the seeds while keeping the bottom intact to create a well for the filling.

3. **Mix the Filling:** In a bowl, combine chopped walnuts, honey or maple syrup, melted coconut oil, ground cinnamon, ground nutmeg, and a pinch of salt. Mix well to create a cohesive filling.

4. **Fill the Apples:** Place the cored apples on a baking dish. Stuff each apple with the prepared filling, ensuring an even distribution.

5. **Bake:** Bake in the preheated oven for approximately 30 minutes or until the apples are tender. The filling should be golden and fragrant.

6. **Serve Warm:** Remove the baked apples from the oven and let them cool for a few minutes. Serve the baked apples warm, either on their own or with a dollop of Greek yogurt or a scoop of vanilla ice cream.

Nutritional Information per serving: Calories: Approximately 250 kcal, Protein: 3g, Fat: 15g, Carbohydrates: 30g, Fiber: 5g, Sugar: 20g, Calcium: 30mg, Iron: 1mg

Dark Chocolate-Dipped Strawberries

Prep Time: 15 minutes | **Cooking Time:** 5 minutes | **Total Time:** 1 hour | **Serving Size:** 4 strawberries

Ingredients:
- 1 pound fresh strawberries, washed and dried
- 8 ounces dark chocolate (at least 70% cocoa), chopped
- 1 tablespoon coconut oil
- Optional toppings: chopped nuts, shredded coconut, or chia seeds

Directions:

1. **Prep the Strawberries:** Wash and thoroughly dry the strawberries. Make sure they are completely dry to help the chocolate adhere better.

2. **Melt the Chocolate:** In a heatproof bowl, combine the chopped dark chocolate and coconut oil.

3.
4. Melt the chocolate using a double boiler or in the microwave at 30-second intervals, stirring until smooth.

5. **Dip the Strawberries:** Hold each strawberry by the stem and dip it into the melted chocolate, ensuring even coverage. Allow any excess chocolate to drip off before placing the dipped strawberry on a parchment paper-lined tray.

6. **Add Toppings (Optional):** While the chocolate is still wet, sprinkle chopped nuts, shredded coconut, or chia seeds on top for added flavor and texture.

7. **Chill:** Place the tray of dipped strawberries in the refrigerator for at least 30 minutes or until the chocolate hardens.

8. **Serve and Enjoy:** Once the chocolate has set, transfer the strawberries to a serving plate. Serve and enjoy these delicious, healthier dark chocolate-dipped strawberries as a delightful dessert or snack.

Nutritional Information per serving: Calories: approximately 120, Fat: 8g, Carbohydrates: 12g, Fiber: 3g, Protein: 2g

Chia Seed Pudding with Fruit

Prep Time: 10 minutes | **Cooking Time:** 0 minutes | **Total Time:** 4 hours | **Serving Size:** 2

Ingredients:

- 1/4 cup chia seeds
- 1 cup almond milk (or any preferred milk)
- 1 tablespoon honey or maple syrup
- 1/2 teaspoon vanilla extract
- A pinch of salt
- Fresh fruits (e.g., berries, kiwi, mango) for topping

Directions:

1. **Mixing the Base:** In a bowl, combine chia seeds, almond milk, honey or maple syrup, vanilla extract, and a pinch of salt. Whisk the ingredients thoroughly to avoid clumps. Let the mixture sit for 5 minutes and then whisk again to prevent chia seeds from settling.

2. **Refrigeration:** Cover the bowl and refrigerate for at least 4 hours or overnight to allow the chia seeds to absorb the liquid and form a pudding-like consistency.

3. **Stirring and Adjustments:** After the initial refrigeration period, give the mixture a good stir to break up any clumps. Taste and adjust sweetness if necessary by adding more honey or maple syrup.

4. **Serving:** Divide the chia seed pudding into serving glasses or bowls.

5. **Fruit Topping:** Wash and chop fresh fruits of your choice. Top each serving of chia pudding with a generous amount of fresh fruits.

6. **Final Touch:** Optionally, drizzle a bit more honey or maple syrup on top for added sweetness.

7. **Enjoy:** Serve chilled and enjoy a healthy, delicious chia seed pudding with a burst of fresh fruit flavors.

Nutritional Information per serving: Calories: 250 | Protein: 8g | Fat: 12g | Carbohydrates: 30g | Fiber: 12g | Sugar: 12g

Greek Yogurt Parfait with Honey and almonds

Prep Time: 10 minutes | **Cook Time:** 0 minutes | **Total Time:** 10 minutes | **Serving Size:** 2 parfaits

Ingredients:

- 1/4 cup honey
- 1/2 cup sliced almonds
- 1 cup mixed berries (blueberries, strawberries, or raspberries)
- 2 cups Greek yogurt (full-fat or low-fat)

Directions:

1. **Prepare Ingredients:** Measure 2 cups of Greek yogurt. Slice almonds and set aside. Wash and prepare the mixed berries.

2. **Layering the Parfait:** Start with a layer of Greek yogurt at the bottom of serving glasses. Add a spoonful of mixed berries on top. Drizzle honey over the berries and yogurt. Sprinkle a layer of sliced almonds.

3. **Repeat Layers:** Repeat the layers until the glass is filled, finishing with a final drizzle of honey and a sprinkle of almonds.

4. **Serve Immediately:** Enjoy the parfait immediately for the best texture and flavor.

Nutritional Information per serving: Calories: Approximately 300, Protein: 20g, Fat: 15g, Carbohydrates: 25g, Fiber: 5g, Sugar: 18g

Frozen Banana Bites

Prep Time: 15 minutes | **Cooking Time:** 0 minutes | **Total Time:** 2 hours | **Serving Size:** 4

Ingredients:

- 3 ripe bananas
- 1/2 cup unsweetened Greek yogurt
- 1 tablespoon honey or maple syrup
- 1/4 cup chopped nuts (almonds, walnuts, or pistachios)
- 1/4 cup shredded unsweetened coconut
- 1/2 teaspoon vanilla extract
- Dark chocolate (optional, for drizzling)

Directions:

1. Peel and slice bananas into bite-sized pieces.
2. Line a baking sheet with parchment paper.
3. In a bowl, mix Greek yogurt, honey or maple syrup, chopped nuts, shredded coconut, and vanilla extract.
4. Dip banana slices into the yogurt mixture, ensuring they're evenly coated.
5. Place the coated banana slices on the prepared baking sheet.
6. After coating the banana slices, place the baking sheet in the freezer for at least 2 hours or until the bites are frozen.
7. If desired, melt dark chocolate and drizzle it over the frozen banana bites for an extra touch (dark chocolate in moderation can have health benefits).
8. Once fully frozen, transfer the banana bites to an airtight container and store in the freezer until ready to serve.

Nutritional Information per serving: Calories: 150, Protein: 4g, Carbohydrates: 25g, Fat: 5g, Fiber: 3g, Sugar: 15g

Avocado Chocolate Mousse

Prep Time: 15 minute | **Cooking Time:** 0 minutes | **Total Time:** 15 minutes | **Serving Size:** 4

Ingredients:

- 2 ripe avocados, peeled and pitted
- 1/3 cup unsweetened cocoa powder
- 1/4 cup almond milk (unsweetened)
- 1/4 cup maple syrup or honey
- 1 teaspoon vanilla extract
- A pinch of salt
- Optional toppings: fresh berries, chopped nuts

Directions:

1. In a food processor or blender, combine the ripe avocados, cocoa powder, almond milk, maple syrup (or honey), vanilla extract, and a pinch of salt.

2. Blend the ingredients until smooth and creamy. If the mixture is too thick, you can add a little more almond milk to achieve the desired consistency.

3. Taste the mousse and adjust sweetness if needed by adding more maple syrup or honey.

4. Once the mixture is smooth and well combined, spoon it into serving bowls or glasses.

5. Refrigerate the mousse for at least 2 hours to allow it to chill and set.

6. Before serving, you can garnish with fresh berries or chopped nuts for added texture and flavor.

7. Enjoy this creamy and indulgent chocolate mousse that is not only delicious but also friendly for those with concerns about fatty liver health.

Nutritional Information per serving: Calories: 180, Total Fat: 12g, Saturated Fat: 2g, Cholesterol: 0mg, Sodium: 20mg, Total Carbohydrates: 20g, Dietary Fiber: 8g, Sugars: 9g, Protein: 3g

Baked Pears with Ricotta and Honey

Prep Time: 15 minutes | **Cook Time:** 25 minutes | **Total Time:** 40 minutes | **Serving Size:** 4

Ingredients:

- 4 ripe pears, halved and cored
- 1 cup ricotta cheese
- 2 tablespoons honey
- 1/4 cup chopped walnuts
- 1 teaspoon vanilla extract
- 1/2 teaspoon cinnamon
- A pinch of salt

Directions:

1. **Preheat the Oven:** Preheat your oven to 375°F (190°C).

2. **Prepare Pears:** Place the halved and cored pears in a baking dish, cut side up.

3. **Ricotta Filling:** In a bowl, mix the ricotta cheese, honey, chopped walnuts, vanilla extract, cinnamon, and a pinch of salt until well combined.

4. **Fill Pears:** Spoon the ricotta mixture evenly into the center of each pear half.

5. **Bake:** Place the baking dish in the preheated oven and bake for 25 minutes or until the pears are tender and the ricotta filling is lightly golden.

6. **Serve:** Once baked, remove from the oven and let it cool slightly. Drizzle additional honey on top if desired.

Nutritional Information per serving: Calories: 220, Total Fat: 10g, Saturated Fat: 5g, Cholesterol: 25mg, Sodium: 80mg, Total Carbohydrates: 30g, Dietary Fiber: 5g, Sugars: 20g, Protein: 7g

Coconut and Berry Ice Pops

Prep Time: 15 minutes | **Cooking Time:** 0 minutes | **Total Time:** 4 hours | **Serving Size:** 6 ice pops

Ingredients:

- 1 cup fresh mixed berries (strawberries, blueberries, raspberries)
- 1 can (14 oz) coconut milk (full fat)
- 2 tablespoons honey or maple syrup (adjust to taste)
- 1 teaspoon vanilla extract

Directions:

1. **Prepare Berries:** Wash and chop the berries into small pieces. Set aside a handful of berries for later use.

2. **Blend Coconut Mixture:** In a blender, combine coconut milk, honey or maple syrup, and vanilla extract. Blend until smooth and well combined.

3. **Layering Ice Pops:** Place a few pieces of chopped berries at the bottom of each ice pop mold. Pour the blended coconut mixture over the berries, filling each mold about halfway.

4. **Adding More Berries:** Add a few more chopped berries into each mold on top of the coconut mixture.

5. **Fill and Freeze:** Top off each mold with the remaining coconut mixture, leaving a little space at the top. Insert ice pop sticks into the molds. Freeze for at least 4 hours or until fully set.

6. **Serve:** Once the ice pops are completely frozen, run the mold under warm water to release them. Serve immediately and enjoy these refreshing and liver-friendly treats!

Nutritional Information per ice pop: Calories: Approximately 120 kcal, **Protein:** 1.5g, **Fat:** 10g, **Carbohydrates:** 8g, **Fiber:** 2g, **Sugar:** 5g, **Sodium:** 10mg

Oatmeal Banana Cookies

Cooking Time: 12-15 minutes | **Prep Time:** 15 minutes | **Total Time:** 30 minutes | **Serving Size:** 2

Ingredients:
- 2 ripe bananas, mashed
- 1 cup rolled oats
- 1/2 cup whole wheat flour
- 1/4 cup coconut oil, melted
- 1/4 cup honey or maple syrup
- 1/2 teaspoon vanilla extract
- 1/2 teaspoon cinnamon
- 1/4 teaspoon salt
- 1/2 cup chopped nuts (such as walnuts or almonds)
- 1/4 cup dark chocolate chips (optional)

Directions:

1. **Preheat the oven:** Preheat your oven to 350°F (175°C). Line a baking sheet with parchment paper.

2. **Mash bananas:** In a large bowl, mash the ripe bananas with a fork until smooth.

3. **Combine wet ingredients:** Add melted coconut oil, honey or maple syrup, and vanilla extract to the mashed bananas. Mix well.

4. **Add dry ingredients:** In the same bowl, add rolled oats, whole wheat flour, cinnamon, and salt. Stir until all ingredients are well combined.

5. **Fold in extras:** Gently fold in the chopped nuts and dark chocolate chips if using.

6. **Form cookies:** Drop spoonful's of the cookie dough onto the prepared baking sheet, spacing them evenly. Flatten each cookie slightly with the back of the spoon.

7. **Bake:** Bake in the preheated oven for 12-15 minutes or until the edges are golden brown.

8. **Cool:** Allow the cookies to cool on the baking sheet for a few minutes before transferring them to a wire rack to cool completely.

Nutritional Information per serving, makes about 12 cookies: Calories: ~120, Protein: 2g, Fat: 6g, Carbohydrates: 16g, Fiber: 2g, Sugar: 6g, Sodium: 50mg

Berry Sorbet

Cooking Time: 12-15 minutes | **Prep Time:** 15 minutes \ **Total Time:** 30 minutes | **Serving Size:** 2

Ingredients:

- 2 ripe bananas, mashed
- 1 cup rolled oats
- 1/2 cup whole wheat flour
- 1/4 cup coconut oil, melted
- 1/4 cup honey or maple syrup
- 1/2 teaspoon vanilla extract
- 1/2 teaspoon cinnamon
- 1/4 teaspoon salt
- 1/2 cup chopped nuts (such as walnuts or almonds)
- 1/4 cup dark chocolate chips (optional)

Directions:

1. **Preheat the oven:** Preheat your oven to 350°F (175°C). Line a baking sheet with parchment paper.

2. **Mash bananas:** In a large bowl, mash the ripe bananas with a fork until smooth.

3. **Combine wet ingredients:** Add melted coconut oil, honey or maple syrup, and vanilla extract to the mashed bananas. Mix well.

4. **Add dry ingredients:** In the same bowl, add rolled oats, whole wheat flour, cinnamon, and salt. Stir until all ingredients are well combined.

5. **Fold in extras:** Gently fold in the chopped nuts and dark chocolate chips if using.

6. **Form cookies:** Drop spoonful's of the cookie dough onto the prepared baking sheet, spacing them evenly. Flatten each cookie slightly with the back of the spoon.

7. **Bake:** Bake in the preheated oven for 12-15 minutes or until the edges are golden brown.

8. **Cool:** Allow the cookies to cool on the baking sheet for a few minutes before transferring them to a wire rack to cool completely.

Nutritional Information per serving: Calories: ~120, Protein: 2g, Fat: 6g, Carbohydrates: 16g, Fiber: 2g, Sugar: 6g, Sodium: 50mg

Grilled Lemon Herb Chicken

Prep Time: 15 minutes | **Cooking Time:** 15 minutes | **Total Time:** 30 minutes | **Servings:** 4

Ingredients:

- 4 boneless, skinless chicken breasts
- 2 lemons (zested and juiced)
- 3 cloves garlic, minced
- 2 tablespoons fresh parsley, chopped
- 1 tablespoon fresh thyme, chopped
- 1 tablespoon fresh rosemary, chopped
- 2 tablespoons olive oil
- Salt and pepper to taste

Directions:

1. **Marinate the Chicken:** In a bowl, combine lemon zest, lemon juice, minced garlic, chopped parsley, thyme, rosemary, olive oil, salt, and pepper. Place the chicken breasts in a zip-top bag or shallow dish and pour the marinade over them. Ensure the chicken is evenly coated. Seal the bag or cover the dish and let it marinate in the refrigerator for at least 30 minutes, allowing the flavors to infuse.

2. **Preheat the Grill:** Preheat your grill to medium-high heat (around 375-400°F or 190-200°C).

3. **Grill the Chicken:** Remove the marinated chicken from the refrigerator and let it come to room temperature for a few minutes. Grease the grill grates to prevent sticking. Grill the chicken breasts for about 6-8 minutes per side or until the internal temperature reaches 165°F (74°C). Baste the chicken with any remaining marinade during grilling for added flavor.

4. **Rest and Serve:** Once cooked, transfer the chicken to a plate and let it rest for a few minutes. This helps rete in juices and ensures a tender result.

5. **Serve and Enjoy:** Slice the grilled lemon herb chicken and serve it with your favorite side dishes, such as roasted vegetables, quinoa, or a leafy green salad.

Nutritional Information (per serving): Calories: Approximately 250 kcal, Protein: 30g, Fat: 12g, Carbohydrates: 5g, Fiber: 2g, Sugar: 1g

Baked Rosemary Turkey Cutlets

Prep Time: 15 minutes | **Cooking Times**: 25 | **Total Time**: 40 minutes **Serving Size**: 1 turkey cutlet

Ingredients:
- 4 turkey cutlets
- 2 tablespoons olive oil
- 1 tablespoon fresh rosemary, chopped
- 2 cloves garlic, minced
- Salt and pepper to taste
- 1 lemon, sliced (optional for garnish)

Directions:

1. **Preparation**: Preheat your oven to 375°F (190°C). Pat dry the turkey cutlets with paper towels to remove excess moisture.

2. **Marinating**: In a small bowl, mix olive oil, chopped rosemary, minced garlic, salt, and pepper to create a marinade. Coat the turkey cutlets evenly with the marinade. Allow them to marinate for at least 15 minutes, or refrigerate for a more intense flavor (up to 24 hours).

3. **Baking**: Place the marinated turkey cutlets on a baking sheet lined with parchment paper. Bake in the preheated oven for approximately 20-25 minutes or until the internal temperature reaches 165°F (74°C), flipping halfway through for even cooking.

4. **Garnish and Serve:** Garnish with fresh rosemary and lemon slices (if desired) before serving. Serve the turkey cutlets with a side of roasted vegetables or a green salad for a well-balanced meal.

Nutritional Information per serving: Calories: Approx. 220, Protein: 25g, Total Fat: 10g, Saturated Fat: 2g, Carbohydrates: 1g, Fiber: 0g, Sugar: 0g, Cholesterol: 70mg, Sodium: 100mg

Lemon Garlic Roast Chicken Thighs

Cooking Time: 35-40 minutes | **Prep Time**: 20 minutes | **Total Time**: 1 hour | **Serving size**: 1

Ingredients:

- 4 bone-in, skin-on chicken thighs
- 2 lemons, juiced and zested
- 4 cloves garlic, minced
- 2 tablespoons olive oil
- 1 teaspoon dried thyme
- 1 teaspoon paprika
- Salt and pepper to taste
- Chopped fresh parsley for garnish (optional)

Directions:

1. **Preparation**: Preheat your oven to 400°F (200°C). Rinse the chicken thighs under cold water and pat them dry with paper towels.

2. **Mari nation**: In a bowl, mix the lemon juice, lemon zest, minced garlic, olive oil, dried thyme, paprika, salt, and pepper to create a marinade. Place the chicken thighs in a shallow dish and coat them evenly with the marinade. Allow the chicken to marinate for at least 30 minutes, or refrigerate for a few hours to enhance flavor.

3. **Cooking**: Place the marinated chicken thighs on a baking sheet lined with parchment paper. Roast in the preheated oven for approximately 35-40 minutes or until the internal temperature reaches 165°F (74°C). For a crispier skin, you can broil for an additional 2-3 minutes, keeping a close eye to prevent burning.

4. **Serve**: Once cooked, remove the chicken from the oven and let it rest for a few minutes before serving. Garnish with chopped fresh parsley if desired.

Nutritional Information per serving: Calories: Approximately 300 kcal, Protein: 25g, Fat: 20g, Carbohydrates: 5g, Fiber: 1g, Sugars: 1g, Sodium: 400mg

Herb-Crusted Baked Chicken Drumsticks

Cooking Time: 20 minutes | **Prep Time**: 10 minutes | **Total Time**: 30 minutes | **Serving size:** 1

Ingredients:
- 8 chicken drumsticks
- 2 tablespoons olive oil
- 1 cup whole wheat breadcrumbs
- 1 tablespoon dried thyme
- 1 tablespoon dried rosemary
- 1 teaspoon garlic powder
- 1 teaspoon onion powder
- Salt and pepper to taste

Directions:

1. **Preheat the Oven**: Preheat your oven to 400°F (200°C).

2. **Prepare the Drumsticks**: Pat dry the chicken drumsticks with paper towels to remove excess moisture Place the drumsticks in a large bowl and drizzle with olive oil. Season with salt and pepper, ensuring even coating.

3. **Prepare Herb Crust:** In a separate bowl, mix breadcrumbs, thyme, rosemary, garlic powder, and onion powder.

4. **Coat Drumsticks:** Roll each drumstick in the herb mixture, ensuring they are evenly coated.

5. **Arrange on Baking Sheet**: Place a wire rack on a baking sheet to allow air circulation. Arrange the coated drumsticks on the rack.

6. **Bake**: Bake in the preheated oven for about 35-40 minutes or until the internal temperature reaches 165°F (74°C) and the crust is golden brown.

7. **Serve**: Allow the chicken to rest for a few minutes before serving.

Nutritional Information: **Serving Size**: 2 drumsticks, **Calories**: Approximately 250 kcal per serving, **Protein**: 30g, **Fat**: 12g, **Carbohydrates**: 8g, **Fiber**: 2g

Sesame Ginger Grilled Chicken Skewers

Cooking Time: 20 minutes | **Prep Time**: 10 minutes | **Total Time**: 30 minutes | **Serving size:** 4

Ingredients:

- 1.5 lbs boneless, skinless chicken breasts, cut into cubes
- 3 tablespoons sesame oil
- 2 tablespoons low-sodium soy sauce
- 1 tablespoon grated fresh ginger
- 2 cloves garlic, minced
- 1 tablespoon honey
- 1 tablespoon rice vinegar
- 1 tablespoon sesame seeds
- Salt and pepper to taste
- Fresh cilantro for garnish (optional)

Directions:

1. **Marinating the Chicken**: In a bowl, combine sesame oil, soy sauce, grated ginger, minced garlic, honey, rice vinegar, sesame seeds, salt, and pepper. Add the chicken cubes to the marinade, ensuring they are well coated. Cover the bowl and refrigerate for at least 30 minutes to allow the flavors to meld.

2. **Skewering the Chicken:** Preheat your grill to medium-high heat. Thread the marinated chicken cubes onto skewers, leaving a little space between each piece for even cooking.

3. **Grilling**: Place the skewers on the preheated grill. Grill for approximately 10-15 minutes, turning occasionally, until the chicken is cooked through and has a nice char.

4. **Serving**: Sprinkle sesame seeds and fresh cilantro on top for extra flavor and presentation. Serve the skewers over a bed of steamed vegetables or a small portion of whole grains like quinoa or brown rice.

Nutritional Information: Nutritional Information: (Per serving) Calories: ~250, Protein: ~30g, Fat: ~10g, Carbohydrates: ~8g.

Baked Parmesan-Crusted Chicken Tenders

Prep Time: 10 minutes | **Cook Time**: 15-20 minutes | **Total Time**: 25-30 minutes | **Serving Size**: 4

Ingredients:

- 1 pound chicken tenders
- 1 cup grated Parmesan cheese
- 1/2 cup almond flour
- 1 teaspoon garlic powder
- 1 teaspoon onion powder
- 1 teaspoon dried oregano
- 1/2 teaspoon salt
- 1/4 teaspoon black pepper
- 2 large eggs

Directions:

1. **Preheat Oven**: Preheat your oven to 400°F (200°C). Line a baking sheet with parchment paper or lightly grease it.

2. **Prepare Coating:** In a shallow bowl, combine Parmesan cheese, almond flour, garlic powder, onion powder, dried oregano, salt, and black pepper. Mix well to create the coating mixture.

3. **Beat Eggs:** In another bowl, beat the eggs. This will be used as a binding agent for the coating.

4. **Coat Chicken Tenders:** Dip each chicken tender into the beaten eggs, ensuring it's fully coated. Then, dredge the chicken in the Parmesan mixture, pressing the coating onto the chicken to adhere.

5. **Place on Baking Sheet:** Arrange the coated chicken tenders on the prepared baking sheet, leaving some space between each piece.

6. **Bake**: Bake in the preheated oven for approximately 15-20 minutes or until the chicken is cooked through and the coating is golden brown. Make sure to flip the tenders halfway through the baking time for even crispiness.

7. **Check Doneness**: To ensure the chicken is fully cooked, use a meat thermometer. The internal temperature should reach 165°F (74°C).

8. **Serve**: Once done, remove the chicken tenders from the oven and let them rest for a few minutes before serving.

Nutritional Information per Serving: Calories: 350, Protein: 35g, Fat: 20g, Carbohydrates: 5g, Fiber: 2g, Sugar: 1g, Sodium: 700mg

Cilantro Lime Grilled Turkey Burgers

Prep Time: 15 minutes | **Cook Time**: 12-15 minutes | **Total Time**: 30 minutes | **Servings**: 4 burgers

Ingredients:

- 1 pound lean ground turkey
- 1/4 cup finely chopped fresh cilantro
- 2 tablespoons fresh lime juice
- 1 teaspoon ground cumin
- 1 teaspoon garlic powder
- 1/2 teaspoon onion powder
- Salt and pepper to taste
- Whole wheat burger buns
- Lettuce, tomato, and onion slices for toppings (optional)

Directions:

1. **Preheat Grill**: Preheat your grill to medium-high heat.

2. **Prepare the Turkey Mix**: In a large mixing bowl, combine ground turkey, chopped cilantro, lime juice, cumin, garlic powder, onion powder, salt, and pepper. Mix thoroughly until all ingredients are evenly distributed.

3. **Shape the Patties**: Divide the turkey mixture into four equal portions and shape them into burger patties. Ensure they are well-formed to prevent falling apart on the grill.

4. **Grill the Burgers**: Place the turkey burgers on the preheated grill. Cook for approximately 6-8 minutes per side, or until the internal temperature reaches 165°F (74°C). Cooking time may vary based on grill temperature.

5. **Toast the Buns:** In the last few minutes of cooking, place the whole wheat burger buns on the grill to lightly toast.

6. **Assemble the Burgers**: Once the turkey burgers are cooked through, place them on the toasted buns. Add lettuce, tomato, and onion slices if desired.

7. **Serve**: Serve the cilantro lime grilled turkey burgers hot. Consider a side salad or grilled vegetables for a complete, liver-friendly meal.

Nutritional Information per serving: Calories: ~250, Protein: ~25g, Fat: ~10g, Carbohydrates: ~15g, Fiber: ~3g, Sugar: ~2g, Sodium: ~300mg

Roasted Garlic and Herb Cornish Hens

Prep Time: 15 minutes | **Cook Time**: 1 hour | **Total Time**: 1 hour and 15 minutes | **Serving Size**: 2

Ingredients:

- 2 Cornish hens
- 4 cloves garlic, minced
- 2 tablespoons olive oil
- 1 teaspoon dried thyme
- 1 teaspoon dried rosemary
- 1 teaspoon dried sage
- Salt and pepper to taste
- 1 lemon, sliced
- Fresh herbs for garnish (optional)

Directions:

1. **Preheat the Oven**: Preheat your oven to 375°F (190°C).
2. **Clean and Pat Dry:** Rinse the Cornish hens under cold water and pat them dry with paper towels. This helps the skin crisp up during roasting.
3. **Season the Hens**: In a small bowl, mix minced garlic, olive oil, dried thyme, rosemary, sage, salt, and pepper to create an herb paste. Rub this mixture all over the hens, making sure to get it under the skin for maximum flavor.

4. **Stuff with Lemon**: Place lemon slices inside the cavity of each hen. This adds a citrusy aroma and keeps the meat moist.

5. **Trusroasting:** Places the Hens (optional): Trussing helps the hens cook evenly. You can use kitchen twine to tie the legs together.

6. The hens in a roasting pan, breast side up. Roast in the preheated oven for about 1 hour or until the internal temperature reaches 165°F (74°C).

7. **Baste Occasionally:** Every 20-30 minutes, baste the hens with the juices in the pan. This adds extra flavor and moisture.

8. **Resting:** Once done, let the hens rest for about 10 minutes before carving. This helps redistribute the juices for juicier meat.

9. **Garnish and Serve:** Garnish with fresh herbs if desired and serve the roasted Cornish hens with your favorite side dishes.

Nutritional Information per serving: Calories: 500, Fat: 30g, Carbohydrates: 2g, Protein: 55g

Mango Salsa Chicken Breasts

Prep Time: 15 minutes | **Cooking Time:** 20 minutes | **Total Time:** 35 minutes | **Serving:** 4

Ingredients:

- 4 boneless, skinless chicken breasts
- 1 ripe mango, diced
- 1/2 red onion, finely chopped
- 1 red bell pepper, diced
- 1 jalapeño, seeds removed and finely chopped
- 2 tablespoons fresh cilantro, chopped
- 2 tablespoons lime juice
- 1 tablespoon olive oil
- Salt and pepper to taste

Directions:

1. **Marinate the Chicken:** Season the chicken breasts with salt and pepper. In a bowl, mix lime juice and olive oil. Brush the chicken breasts with the lime and olive oil mixture. Let them marinate for 10 minutes.

2. **Preheat the Grill or Pan:** Preheat your grill or a non-stick pan over medium-high heat.

3. **Grill the Chicken:** Place the marinated chicken breasts on the preheated grill or pan. Cook for approximately 8-10 minutes per side or until the internal temperature reaches 165°F (74°C).

4. **Prepare the Mango Salsa:** In a separate bowl, combine diced mango, red onion, red bell pepper, jalapeño, and cilantro. Add salt to taste and mix well.

5. **Serve:** Once the chicken is cooked thoroughly, remove it from the grill or pan. Top each chicken breast with a generous portion of mango salsa.

6. **Enjoy:** Serve the Mango Salsa Chicken Breasts with a side of steamed vegetables or a green salad for a wholesome, liver-friendly meal.

Nutritional Information per serving: Calories: 250, Protein: 30g, Carbohydrates: 15g, Fat: 8g, Fiber: 3g

Greek Yogurt Marinated Chicken Kebabs

Prep Time: 10 minutes | **Cooking Time:** 2 hours | **Total Time:** 2 hours| **Serving:** 4

Ingredients:

- 1.5 lbs boneless, skinless chicken breasts, cut into chunks
- 1 cup Greek yogurt
- 3 tablespoons olive oil
- 4 cloves garlic, minced
- 1 tablespoon fresh lemon juice
- 1 teaspoon dried oregano
- 1 teaspoon ground cumin
- 1 teaspoon paprika
- Salt and pepper to taste
- Wooden skewers, soaked in water for 30 minutes

Directions:

1. **Marinate the Chicken:** In a bowl, mix Greek yogurt, olive oil, minced garlic, lemon juice, oregano, cumin, paprika, salt, and pepper to create the marinade. Add the chicken chunks to the marinade, ensuring they are well-coated. Cover the bowl and refrigerate for at least 2 hours or overnight for optimal flavor.

2. **Preparation:** Preheat your grill to medium-high heat.

3. **Skewering:** Thread marinated chicken chunks onto the soaked wooden skewers, leaving a little space between each piece.

4. **Grilling:** Place the skewers on the preheated grill and cook for about 12-15 minutes, turning occasionally, until the chicken is fully cooked and has a nice char.

5. **Check for Doneness:** Ensure the chicken reaches an internal temperature of 165°F (74°C).

6. **Serve:** Remove the kebabs from the grill and let them rest for a few minutes.

7. **Serving Size:** This recipe serves approximately 4 people.

8. **Enjoy:** Serve the Greek Yogurt Marinated Chicken Kebabs with a side of roasted vegetables or a fresh salad.

Nutritional Information Per serving: Calories: 250, Protein: 30g, Fat: 12g, Carbohydrates: 5g, Fiber: 1g.

<h1 style="text-align:center">FISH AND SEAFOOD</h1>

Baked Lemon Garlic Salmon

Prep Time: 10 minutes | **Cook Time:** 15-20 minutes | **Total Time:** 30 minutes | **Serving Size:** 1 fillet

Ingredients:
- 4 salmon fillets (about 6 ounces each)
- 2 tablespoons olive oil
- 3 cloves garlic, minced
- 1 teaspoon dried oregano
- 1 teaspoon dried thyme
- Salt and pepper to taste
- Zest of 1 lemon
- Juice of 1 lemon
- Fresh parsley for garnish

Directions:

1. **Preheat Oven:** Preheat your oven to 375°F (190°C).

2. **Prepare Salmon:** Pat the salmon fillets dry with paper towels. Place them on a baking sheet lined with parchment paper.

3. **Seasoning Mix:** In a small bowl, mix olive oil, minced garlic, dried oregano, dried thyme, salt, and pepper.

4. **Coat Salmon:** Brush the salmon fillets with the prepared seasoning mix, making sure to coat them evenly.

5. **Lemon Zest and Juice:** Sprinkle lemon zest over the fillets and drizzle lemon juice on top for a burst of citrus flavor.

6. **Bake:** Bake the salmon in the preheated oven for about 15-20 minutes, or until the salmon flakes easily with a fork. Cooking time may vary based on the thickness of the fillets.

7. **Garnish:** Once done, remove from the oven and garnish with fresh parsley for a vibrant finish.

8. **Serve:** Serve the Baked Lemon Garlic Salmon hot, paired with your favorite steamed vegetables or a side salad.

Nutritional Information: Calories: Approximately 300 per serving, Protein: 35g, Fat: 16g, Carbohydrates: 2g, Fiber: 1g

Grilled Herb-Infused Tilapia

Prep Time: 15 minutes | **Cooking Time:** 10 minutes | **Total Time:** 25 minutes | **Serving Size:** 4

Ingredients:

- 4 tilapia fillets
- 2 tablespoons olive oil
- 1 teaspoon dried thyme
- 1 teaspoon dried oregano
- 1 teaspoon dried rosemary
- 1 teaspoon garlic powder
- Salt and pepper to taste
- Lemon wedges for serving

Directions:

1. **Preheat the Grill:** Preheat your grill to medium-high heat.

2. **Prepare the Tilapia:** Pat the tilapia fillets dry with paper towels. In a small bowl, mix together the olive oil, dried thyme, dried oregano, dried rosemary, garlic powder, salt, and pepper to create the herb-infused marinade.

3. **Marinate the Tilapia:** Brush both sides of the tilapia fillets with the herb-infused marinade, ensuring they are well coated. Allow the fillets to marinate for at least 10 minutes, letting the flavors infuse into the fish.

4. **Grill the Tilapia:** Place the marinated tilapia fillets on the preheated grill. Grill for approximately 4-5 minutes per side, or until the fish is opaque and easily flakes with a fork.

5. **Serve:** Carefully remove the grilled tilapia from the grill. Serve the tilapia hot, garnished with lemon wedges on the side.

6. **Enjoy:** Delight in this flavorful and heart-healthy grilled tilapia, rich in omega-3 fatty acids and low in saturated fat.

Nutritional Information per serving: Calories: 200, Protein: 25g, Fat: 10g, Carbohydrates: 1g, Fiber: 0g, Sugar: 0g, Cholesterol: 60mg, Sodium: 150mg

Miso-Glazed Cod

Prep Time: 15 minutes | **Cooking Time:** 1-2 minutes | **Total Time:** 20 minutes | **Serving Size:** 1

Ingredients:
- 4 cod fillets (about 6 ounces each)
- 1/4 cup white miso paste
- 2 tablespoons miring
- 2 tablespoons sake
- 1 tablespoon reduced-sodium soy sauce
- 1 tablespoon honey or maple syrup
- 1 teaspoon grated ginger
- 2 cloves garlic, minced
- 1 tablespoon sesame oil
- Sesame seeds and sliced green onions for garnish

Directions:

1. **Preparation:** Pat the cod fillets dry with paper towels. In a bowl, whisk together miso paste, miring, sake, soy sauce, honey or maple syrup, grated ginger, and minced garlic to create the glaze.

2. **Marinating:** Place the cod fillets in a shallow dish or resealable plastic bag. Pour half of the miso glaze over the fish, ensuring it's well-coated. Marinate in the refrigerator for at least 30 minutes, turning the fillets halfway through.

3. **Cooking:** Preheat your oven to 400°F (200°C). Heat sesame oil in an oven-safe skillet over medium-high heat. Sear the cod fillets for 1-2 minutes on each side until golden brown. Brush the remaining miso glaze over the fillets.

4. **Baking:** Transfer the skillet to the preheated oven. Bake for 10-12 minutes or until the cod is cooked through and flakes easily with a fork.

5. **Garnish and Serve:** Remove from the oven and garnish with sesame seeds and sliced green onions. Serve the Miso-Glazed Cod over a bed of steamed vegetables or brown rice.

Nutritional Information per Serving: Calories: Approximately 250, Protein: 30g, Total Fat: 8g, Carbohydrates: 10g, Fiber: 1g, Sugars: 5g, Sodium: 600mg

Seared Tuna Steaks with Sesame Seeds

Prep Time: 15 minutes | **Cooking Time:** 6-8 minutes | **Total Time:** 25 minutes | **Serving Size:** 4

Ingredients:

- 4 tuna steaks (about 6 ounces each)
- 2 tablespoons soy sauce (low-sodium if possible)
- 1 tablespoon sesame oil
- 2 tablespoons sesame seeds
- 1 tablespoon olive oil
- 2 cloves garlic, minced
- 1 tablespoon fresh ginger, grated
- Salt and pepper to taste
- Green onions, sliced (for garnish)

Directions:

1. Pat the tuna steaks dry with paper towels.
2. In a shallow dish, mix soy sauce, sesame oil, garlic, and ginger. Place the tuna steaks in the marinade, ensuring they are well-coated. Allow to marinate for at least 10 minutes.
3. Heat olive oil in a skillet over medium-high heat.
4. While the pan is heating, sprinkle sesame seeds on a plate. Press each side of the tuna steaks into the sesame seeds, coating them evenly.
5. Place the tuna steaks in the hot skillet and sear for about 3-4 minutes per side for medium-rare. Adjust the time based on your desired doneness.
6. Transfer the seared tuna steaks to a cutting board and let them rest for a few minutes before slicing.
7. Slice the tuna steaks into 1/2-inch thick slices.
8. Drizzle any remaining marinade over the sliced tuna.
9. Garnish with sliced green onions.

Nutritional Information per serving: Calories: approximately 300, Protein: 30g, Fat: 18g, Carbohydrates: 2g, Fiber: 1g, Sugars: 0g, Cholesterol: 45mg, Sodium: 450mg

Garlic Butter Shrimp Skewers

Prep Time: 15 minutes | **Cook Time:** 6-8 minutes | **Total Time:** 25 minutes

Ingredients:

- 1 pound large shrimp, peeled and deveined
- 3 tablespoons unsalted butter, melted
- 4 cloves garlic, minced
- 1 tablespoon fresh parsley, chopped
- 1 tablespoon lemon juice
- Salt and pepper to taste
- Wooden skewers, soaked in water for 30 minutes

Directions:

1. **Marinating Shrimp:** In a bowl, combine melted butter, minced garlic, chopped parsley, lemon juice, salt, and pepper. Add cleaned shrimp to the marinade, ensuring they are well-coated. Let it marinate in the refrigerator for at least 10 minutes.

2. **Skewering:** Preheat the grill or grill pan over medium heat. Thread the marinated shrimp onto the soaked wooden skewers.

3. **Grilling:** Place the skewers on the preheated grill and cook for 3-4 minutes on each side or until the shrimp are opaque and cooked through. Baste the shrimp with any remaining garlic butter marinade during grilling.

4. **Serve:** Once cooked, remove the shrimp skewers from the grill. Optionally, garnish with additional chopped parsley and serve hot.

Nutritional Information per serving: Calories: Approximately 250, Protein: 25g, Fat: 15g, Carbohydrates: 2g, Fiber: 0.5g, Sugar: 0.5g, Cholesterol: 180mg, Sodium: 300mg

Baked Dijon Mustard Haddock

Prep Time: 15 minutes | **Cooking Time:** 25 minutes | **Total Time:** 40 minutes | **Serving Size:** 4

Ingredients:

- 4 haddock fillets (about 6 ounces each)
- 2 tablespoons Dijon mustard
- 2 tablespoons olive oil
- 1 tablespoon lemon juice
- 2 cloves garlic, minced
- 1 teaspoon dried thyme
- Salt and pepper to taste
- Fresh parsley for garnish

Directions:

1. Preheat your oven to 375°F (190°C).
2. Line a baking dish with parchment paper or lightly grease it.
3. In a small bowl, mix together Dijon mustard, olive oil, lemon juice, minced garlic, dried thyme, salt, and pepper.
4. Place the haddock fillets in the prepared baking dish and brush the mustard mixture evenly over each fillet.
5. Allow the fish to marinate for about 10 minutes.
6. Bake the haddock in the preheated oven for 15-20 minutes or until the fish is opaque and flakes easily with a fork.
7. The cooking time may vary slightly depending on the thickness of the fillets.
8. Once baked, garnish the haddock with fresh parsley.
9. Serve the Baked Dijon Mustard Haddock hot, accompanied by your choice of side dishes like steamed vegetables or a green salad.

Nutritional Information per serving: Calories: 220, Total Fat: 10g, Saturated Fat: 1.5g, Cholesterol: 80mg, Sodium: 300mg, Total Carbohydrates: 2g, Dietary Fiber: 0.5g, Sugars: 0.5g, Protein: 28

Lemon Herb Grilled Swordfish

Prep Time: 15 minutes | **Cooking Time:** 8-10 minutes | **Total Time:** 1 hour | **Serving Size:** 1 swordfish

Ingredients:

- 4 swordfish steaks (about 6 ounces each)
- 1/4 cup fresh lemon juice
- 2 tablespoons olive oil
- 2 cloves garlic, minced
- 1 teaspoon dried oregano
- 1 teaspoon dried thyme
- 1 teaspoon dried rosemary
- Salt and pepper to taste
- Lemon wedges for garnish

Directions:

1. Pat dry the swordfish steaks with paper towels.
2. In a small bowl, whisk together lemon juice, olive oil, minced garlic, oregano, thyme, rosemary, salt, and pepper.
3. Place the swordfish steaks in a shallow dish and pour the marinade over them. Ensure the steaks are well-coated. Let them marinate in the refrigerator for at least 30 minutes.
4. Preheat your grill to medium-high heat. Clean and oil the grates to prevent sticking.
5. Remove the swordfish from the marinade, allowing excess to drip off. Discard the marinade.
6. Grill the swordfish for 4-5 minutes per side, or until the internal temperature reaches 145°F (63°C). The fish should be opaque and easily flaked with a fork.
7. Allow the grilled swordfish to rest for 5 minutes before serving. This helps retain juices and ensures a flavorful, moist result.
8. Garnish with lemon wedges and fresh herbs if desired.
9. Serve the Lemon Herb Grilled Swordfish with a side of steamed vegetables or a green salad for a well-balanced, liver-friendly meal.

Cajun Spiced Catfish Fillets

Prep Time: 10 minutes | **Cooking Time:** 15 minutes | **Total Time**: 25 minutes | **Serving Size:** 4

Ingredients:

- 4 catfish fillets (about 6 ounces each)
- 2 tablespoons olive oil
- 1 tablespoon Cajun seasoning (low-sodium)
- 1 teaspoon garlic powder
- 1 teaspoon onion powder
- 1/2 teaspoon paprika
- 1/2 teaspoon dried thyme
- 1/2 teaspoon dried oregano
- Salt and black pepper to taste
- Fresh lemon wedges for serving

Directions:

1. **Preheat Oven:** Preheat your oven to 375°F (190°C).

2. **Prepare Catfish Fillets:** Pat the catfish fillets dry with paper towels. Place them on a baking sheet lined with parchment paper.

3. **Seasoning Mix:** In a small bowl, mix Cajun seasoning, garlic powder, onion powder, paprika, dried thyme, dried oregano, salt, and black pepper.

4. **Season Catfish:** Brush each catfish fillet with olive oil. Sprinkle the seasoning mix evenly over both sides of each fillet, pressing it gently to adhere.

5. **Bake:** Bake the catfish in the preheated oven for about 12-15 minutes or until the fish flakes easily with a fork.

6. **Serve:** Remove the catfish fillets from the oven and let them rest for a few minutes. Serve hot with fresh lemon wedges on the side.

Nutritional Information per serving: Calories: 250, Total Fat: 12g, Saturated Fat: 2g, Cholesterol: 80mg, Sodium: 300mg, Total Carbohydrates: 2g, Dietary Fiber: 1g, Protein: 30g

Cilantro Lime Shrimp Stir-Fry

Prep Time: 15 minutes | **Cook Time:** 10 minutes | **Total Time:** 25 minutes | **Serving Size:** 4

Ingredients:

- 1 pound shrimp, peeled and deveined
- 2 tablespoons olive oil
- 3 cloves garlic, minced
- 1 tablespoon ginger, grated
- 1 red bell pepper, thinly sliced
- 1 cup sugar snap peas, ends trimmed
- 1 tablespoon low-sodium soy sauce
- 1 tablespoon fish sauce
- 2 teaspoons honey
- Juice of 2 limes
- Salt and pepper to taste
- Fresh cilantro for garnish

Directions:

1. **Marinate Shrimp:** In a bowl, combine shrimp with half of the minced garlic, ginger, lime juice, and a pinch of salt. Let it marinate for 10 minutes.

2. **Prepare Vegetables:** Heat olive oil in a large skillet or wok over medium-high heat. Add the remaining garlic and sauté for 30 seconds. Add sliced bell pepper and sugar snap peas, stir-frying until vegetables are crisp-tender.

3. **Cook Shrimp:** Push the vegetables to the side of the skillet and add the marinated shrimp. Cook for 2-3 minutes on each side until they turn pink and opaque.

4. **Create Sauce:** In a small bowl, whisk together soy sauce, fish sauce, honey, and the remaining lime juice. Pour the sauce over the shrimp and vegetables, tossing everything together.

5. **Adjust Seasoning:** Season with salt and pepper to taste. Adjust the sweetness or acidity by adding more honey or lime juice if desired.

6. **Garnish and Serve:** Sprinkle fresh cilantro over the stir-fry for a burst of flavor and color. Serve the Cilantro Lime Shrimp Stir-Fry over brown rice or cauliflower rice for a liver-friendly option.

Nutritional Information per serving: Calories: 220, Protein: 25g, Fat: 10g, Carbohydrates: 8g, Fiber: 2g

Baked Garlic Parmesan Halibut

Prep Time: 10 minutes | **Cooking Time:** 12-15 minutes | **Total Time:** 25 minutes | **Serving Size:** 4

Ingredients:

- 4 halibut fillets (about 6 ounces each)
- 1/2 cup grated Parmesan cheese
- 2 tablespoons melted butter
- 3 cloves garlic, minced
- 1 teaspoon dried oregano
- 1 teaspoon dried parsley
- 1/2 teaspoon black pepper
- 1/4 teaspoon salt
- Lemon wedges for serving

Directions:

1. **Preheat Oven:** Preheat your oven to 400°F (200°C). Line a baking sheet with parchment paper for easy cleanup.

2. **Prepare Halibut:** Pat the halibut fillets dry with paper towels. Place them on the prepared baking sheet.

3. **Mix Parmesan Mixture:** In a small bowl, combine the grated Parmesan cheese, melted butter, minced garlic, dried oregano, dried parsley, black pepper, and salt. Mix until well combined.

4. **Coat Halibut:** Brush the top side of each halibut fillet with the Parmesan mixture, ensuring an even coating.

5. **Bake:** Bake in the preheated oven for 12-15 minutes or until the halibut is opaque and flakes easily with a fork. The Parmesan topping should be golden and slightly crispy.

6. **Serve:** Remove from the oven and let it rest for a couple of minutes. Serve the Baked Garlic Parmesan Halibut with lemon wedges for a fresh burst of flavor.

Nutritional Information per Serving: Calories: 300, Total Fat: 15g, Saturated Fat: 8g, Cholesterol: 90mg, Sodium: 400mg, Protein: 35g

Quinoa and Black Bean Stuffed Peppers

Prep Time: 20 minutes | **Cooking Time:** 30 minutes | **Total Time:** 50 minutes | **Servings:** 4

Ingredients:

- 4 large bell peppers (any color)
- 1 cup quinoa, rinsed
- 2 cups vegetable broth
- 1 can (15 oz) black beans, drained and rinsed
- 1 cup corn kernels (fresh or frozen)
- 1 cup diced tomatoes
- 1 cup diced red onion
- 2 cloves garlic, minced
- 1 teaspoon ground cumin
- 1 teaspoon chili powder
- Salt and pepper to taste
- 1 cup shredded cheese (optional, for topping)
- Fresh cilantro, chopped (for garnish)

Directions:

1. **Preheat the oven:** Preheat your oven to 375°F (190°C).

2. **Prepare the peppers:** Cut the tops off the bell peppers and remove the seeds and membranes. Lightly brush the outside of each pepper with olive oil and place them in a baking dish.

3. **Cook the quinoa:** In a medium saucepan, combine the rinsed quinoa and vegetable broth. Bring to a boil, then reduce the heat, cover, and simmer for about 15 minutes or until the quinoa is cooked and the liquid is absorbed.

4. **Prepare the filling:** In a large bowl, mix together the cooked quinoa, black beans, corn, diced tomatoes, red onion, minced garlic, cumin, chili powder, salt, and pepper.

5. **Stuff the peppers:** Stuff each bell pepper with the quinoa and black bean mixture, pressing it down gently.

6. **Bake:** Cover the baking dish with foil and bake in the preheated oven for 25-30 minutes or until the peppers are tender.

7. **Optional topping:** If desired, sprinkle shredded cheese on top of each stuffed pepper during the last 5 minutes of baking until melted and bubbly.

8. **Serve:** Remove from the oven and let them cool slightly. Garnish with fresh chopped cilantro.

Nutritional Information per serving: Calories: 350, Total Fat: 5g, Saturated Fat: 2g, Cholesterol: 10mg, Sodium: 600mg, Total Carbohydrates: 65g, Dietary Fiber: 12g, Sugars: 8g, Protein: 14g

Mushroom and Spinach Lentil Loaf

Prep Time: 20 minutes | **Cooking Time:** 1 hour | **Total Time:** 1 hour 20 minutes | **Serving Size:** 6-8

Ingredients:

- 1 cup dry green lentils, rinsed
- 2 1/2 cups vegetable broth
- 2 tablespoons olive oil
- 1 large onion, finely chopped
- 3 cloves garlic, minced
- 8 oz mushrooms, finely chopped
- 2 cups fresh spinach, chopped
- 1 cup rolled oats
- 1/2 cup breadcrumbs
- 1/4 cup ground flaxseed mixed with 1/2 cup water (flax egg)
- 2 tablespoons tomato paste
- 1 tablespoon soy sauce
- 1 teaspoon dried thyme
- 1 teaspoon dried oregano
- Salt and pepper to taste

Directions:

1. **Cook Lentils:** In a medium saucepan, combine lentils and vegetable broth. Bring to a boil, then reduce heat, cover, and simmer for about 25-30 minutes or until lentils are tender. Drain any excess liquid.

2. **Prepare Flax Egg:** In a small bowl, mix ground flaxseed with water and let it sit for 5 minutes until it forms a gel-like consistency.

3. **Sauté Vegetables:** In a large skillet, heat olive oil over medium heat. Add chopped onions and garlic, sauté until translucent. Add mushrooms and cook until they release their moisture. Stir in chopped spinach and cook until wilted.

4. **Combine Ingredients:** In a large mixing bowl, combine cooked lentils, sautéed vegetables, rolled oats, breadcrumbs, flax egg, tomato paste, soy sauce, thyme, oregano, salt, and pepper. Mix well until everything is evenly combined.

5. **Bake:** Preheat the oven to 350°F (175°C). Transfer the mixture to a greased loaf pan, pressing it down firmly. Bake for 40-45 minutes or until the top is golden brown and the edges pull away from the sides.

6. **Cool and Serve:** Allow the lentil loaf to cool in the pan for 10-15 minutes before slicing. Serve slices with your favorite side dishes.

Nutritional Information per serving, based on 6 servings: Calories: ~280, Protein: ~15g, Fat: ~8g, Carbohydrates: ~40g, Fiber: ~10g, Sugars: ~4g

Eggplant and Chickpea Curry

Prep Time: 15 minutes | **Cooking Time:** 30 minutes | **Total Time:** 45 minutes | **Serving Size:** 4

Ingredients:

- 1 large eggplant, diced
- 1 can (15 oz) chickpeas, drained and rinsed
- 1 large onion, finely chopped
- 3 cloves garlic, minced
- 1-inch ginger, grated
- 2 tomatoes, chopped
- 1/2 cup tomato puree
- 1 cup vegetable broth
- 2 tablespoons olive oil
- 1 teaspoon cumin seeds
- 1 teaspoon coriander powder
- 1 teaspoon turmeric powder
- 1 teaspoon garam masala
- 1/2 teaspoon red chili powder (adjust to taste)
- Salt to taste
- Fresh cilantro for garnish

Directions:

1. **Preparation:** Dice the eggplant into bite-sized pieces. Finely chop the onion, mince the garlic, and grate the ginger. Chop the tomatoes and set aside.

2. **Cooking:** Heat olive oil in a large pan over medium heat. Add cumin seeds and let them splutter. Add chopped onions and sauté until golden brown. Add minced garlic and grated ginger, sauté for another minute until fragrant. Stir in coriander powder, turmeric powder, red chili powder, and salt. Cook for 2 minutes. Add chopped tomatoes and cook until they soften. Add tomato puree and cook for an additional 2 minutes.

3. **Adding Vegetables:** Add diced eggplant and chickpeas to the pan. Mix well to coat them with the spices. Pour in the vegetable broth, cover, and simmer for 15-20 minutes until the eggplant is tender.

4. **Finishing Touch:** Sprinkle garam masala over the curry and stir gently. Adjust salt and spice levels according to taste.

5. **Garnish and Serve:** Garnish the curry with fresh cilantro. Serve hot over steamed brown rice or with whole-grain naan.

Nutritional Information per serving: Calories: 300, Fat: 10g, Carbohydrates: 45g, Protein: 12g, Fiber: 10g

Sweet Potato and Kale Buddha Bowl

Prep Time: 15 minutes | **Cook Time:** 45 minutes | **Total Time:** 1 hour | **Serving size**: 1

Ingredients:

- 2 medium-sized sweet potatoes, peeled and cubed
- 1 bunch of kale, stems removed and leaves torn into bite-sized pieces
- 1 cup quinoa, rinsed
- 1 can (15 oz) chickpeas, drained and rinsed
- 1 avocado, sliced
- 1/4 cup pumpkin seeds (optional, for garnish)
- Olive oil for cooking
- Salt and pepper to taste

For the Dressing:

- 3 tablespoons olive oil
- 2 tablespoons apple cider vinegar
- 1 tablespoon maple syrup
- 1 teaspoon Dijon mustard
- Salt and pepper to taste

Directions:

1. Preheat your oven to 400°F (200°C).
2. Toss the cubed sweet potatoes with olive oil, salt, and pepper.
3. Spread them on a baking sheet and roast for 25-30 minutes or until tender and golden brown.
4. In a saucepan, combine quinoa with double the amount of water.
5. Bring to a boil, then reduce heat, cover, and simmer for 15 minutes or until quinoa is cooked and water is absorbed.
6. In a large bowl, massage the torn kale leaves with a bit of olive oil until they become tender.
7. Toss chickpeas with olive oil, salt, and pepper.
8. Spread them on a baking sheet and roast for 20-25 minutes or until crispy.
9. Whisk together olive oil, apple cider vinegar, maple syrup, Dijon mustard, salt, and pepper in a small bowl.
10. In serving bowls, arrange cooked quinoa, roasted sweet potatoes, massaged kale, roasted chickpeas, and sliced avocado.
11. Drizzle the dressing over the bowls, ensuring an even coating.
12. Garnish with pumpkin seeds if desired.
13. Serve immediately, and enjoy this nutrient-rich Buddha Bowl.

Nutritional Information: Calories: Approx. 500, Protein: 15g, Fat: 20g, Carbohydrates: 65g, Fiber: 12g, Sugar: 8g

Zucchini Noodles with Pesto and Cherry Tomatoes

Prep Time: 15 minutes | **Cook Time:** 5 minutes | **Total Time:** 20 minutes | **Serving size**: 2

Ingredients:

- 4 medium-sized zucchini, spiralized into noodles
- 1 cup cherry tomatoes, halved

For Pesto:
- 2 cups fresh basil leaves, packed
- 1/2 cup walnuts or pine nuts
- 1/2 cup grated Parmesan cheese
- 2 garlic cloves, minced
- 1/2 cup extra-virgin olive oil
- Salt and pepper to taste

Directions:

1. **Prepare Pesto:**
   a. In a food processor, combine basil, nuts, Parmesan, and garlic.
   b. Pulse until coarsely chopped.
   c. With the processor running, slowly add olive oil until the mixture is smooth.
   d. Season with salt and pepper to taste.

2. **Cook Zucchini Noodles:**
   a. Spiralize the zucchini into noodles using a spiralizer.
   b. In a large pan, heat a bit of olive oil over medium heat.
   c. Add zucchini noodles and sauté for 2-3 minutes until just tender. Avoid overcooking to maintain a slight crunch.

3. **Combine with Pesto:**
   a. Add the prepared pesto to the zucchini noodles.
   b. Toss until the noodles are well coated with the pesto sauce.

4. **Add Cherry Tomatoes:**
   a. Gently fold in the halved cherry tomatoes to the zucchini and pesto mixture.
   b. Heat for an additional 1-2 minutes until the tomatoes are warmed through but still retain their shape.

5. **Serve:**
   a. Divide the zucchini noodle mixture into serving plates.

Nutritional Information: Calories: Approximately 300 calories per serving, Fat: 25g, Carbohydrates: 10g, Protein: 8g

Cauliflower and Chickpea Tacos

Prep Time: 15 minutes | **Cooking Time:** 25 minutes | **Total Time:** 40 minutes | **Serving Size:** 4.

Ingredients:

- 1 medium cauliflower, cut into small florets
- 1 can (15 oz) chickpeas, drained and rinsed
- 2 tablespoons olive oil
- 1 teaspoon ground cumin
- 1 teaspoon smoked paprika
- 1/2 teaspoon garlic powder
- Salt and pepper to taste
- 8 whole-grain tortillas
- 1 cup shredded red cabbage
- 1 avocado, sliced
- Fresh cilantro, for garnish
- Lime wedges, for serving

Directions:

1. **Preheat Oven:**
   Preheat the oven to 400°F (200°C).

2. **Prepare Vegetables:**
   Toss cauliflower florets and chickpeas in a bowl with olive oil, cumin, smoked paprika, garlic powder, salt, and pepper.

3. **Roast:**
   Spread the seasoned cauliflower and chickpeas on a baking sheet. Roast in the preheated oven for 20-25 minutes or until cauliflower is golden brown and chickpeas are crispy.

4. **Warm Tortillas:**
   While the veggies are roasting, warm the tortillas in a dry skillet or microwave according to package instructions.

5. **Assemble Tacos:**
   Place a spoonful of the roasted cauliflower and chickpeas onto each tortilla. Top with shredded red cabbage, avocado slices, and fresh cilantro.

6. **Serve:**
   Serve the tacos with lime wedges on the side for squeezing.

Nutritional Information per serving: Calories: 300, Protein: 8g, Fat: 10g, Carbohydrates: 45g, Fiber: 10g, Sugar: 5g, Sodium: 350mg

Lentil and Vegetable Stir-Fry

Prep Time: 15 minutes | **Cooking Time:** 25 minutes | **Total Time:** 40 minutes | **Serving Size:** 4

Ingredients:

- 1 cup dry green or brown lentils
- 2 cups mixed vegetables (e.g., broccoli, bell peppers, carrots)
- 1 onion, thinly sliced
- 2 cloves garlic, minced
- 1 tablespoon olive oil
- 1 tablespoon low-sodium soy sauce
- 1 teaspoon sesame oil
- 1 teaspoon ginger, grated
- 1/2 teaspoon turmeric powder
- Salt and pepper to taste
- Fresh cilantro for garnish (optional)

Directions:

1. **Prepare Lentils:** Rinse lentils under cold water. Cook them according to package instructions until tender. Set aside.
2. **Prepare Vegetables:** Chop the mixed vegetables into bite-sized pieces.
3. **Stir-Fry Base:** Heat olive oil in a large skillet or wok over medium heat. Add sliced onions and minced garlic. Sauté until onions are translucent.
4. **Add Vegetables:** Add mixed vegetables to the skillet. Stir-fry for about 5-7 minutes until they are tender-crisp.
5. **Seasoning:** Add soy sauce, sesame oil, grated ginger, turmeric powder, salt, and pepper. Mix well to coat the vegetables evenly.
6. **Incorporate Lentils:** Gently fold in the cooked lentils. Continue cooking for an additional 3-5 minutes until everything is well combined and heated through.
7. **Adjust Seasoning:** Taste and adjust the seasoning if necessary. You can add more soy sauce or salt according to your preference.
8. **Serve:** Garnish with fresh cilantro if desired. Serve the Lentil and Vegetable Stir-Fry over brown rice or quinoa for a wholesome meal.

Nutritional Information per serving: Calories: 250, Protein: 15g, Carbohydrates: 35g, Fiber: 10g, Fat: 6g, Saturated Fat: 1g, Cholesterol: 0mg, Sodium: 300mg

Stuffed Portobello Mushrooms with Quinoa and Kale

Prep Time: 15 minutes | **Cooking Time:** 25 minutes | **Total Time:** 40 minutes | **Serving Size:** 1

Ingredients:

- 4 large Portobello mushrooms, stems removed
- 1 cup quinoa, rinsed
- 2 cups kale, finely chopped
- 1 small onion, finely chopped
- 2 cloves garlic, minced
- 1 tablespoon olive oil
- 1 teaspoon dried oregano
- 1 teaspoon dried thyme
- Salt and pepper to taste
- 1/2 cup crumbled feta cheese (optional)
- Fresh parsley for garnish

Directions:

1. **Preparation:** Preheat your oven to 375°F (190°C). Cook the quinoa according to package instructions. Clean the Portobello mushrooms and remove the stems. Lightly scrape out the gills to create more space for the stuffing.

2. **Sauté the Vegetables:** In a pan, heat olive oil over medium heat. Add chopped onions and garlic, sauté until translucent. Add chopped kale and cook until wilted. Season with salt, pepper, dried oregano, and thyme.

3. **Prepare the Filling:** In a mixing bowl, combine cooked quinoa with the sautéed vegetables. Mix well. If desired, fold in crumbled feta cheese for added flavor.

4. **Stuff the Mushrooms:** Place the Portobello mushrooms on a baking sheet lined with parchment paper. Stuff each mushroom with the quinoa and kale mixture, pressing it down gently.

5. **Bake:** Bake in the preheated oven for 20-25 minutes or until the mushrooms are tender and the filling is heated through.

6. **Serve:** Garnish with fresh parsley before serving.
   - Consider drizzling with a bit of olive oil or balsamic glaze for extra flavor.

Nutritional Information: Calories: 150 kcal, Protein: 7g, Carbohydrates: 25g, Fat: 3g, Fiber: 4g

Chickpea and Sweet Potato Curry

Prep Time: 15 minutes | **Cook Time:** 30 minutes | **Total Time:** 45 minutes | **Servings:** 4

Ingredients:

- 1 cup dried chickpeas, soaked overnight (or use canned, rinsed and drained)
- 2 medium sweet potatoes, peeled and diced
- 1 large onion, finely chopped
- 2 cloves garlic, minced
- 1 tablespoon fresh ginger, grated
- 1 can (14 oz) diced tomatoes
- 1 can (14 oz) coconut milk (light for a lower-fat option)
- 1 tablespoon curry powder
- 1 teaspoon ground cumin
- 1 teaspoon ground coriander
- 1/2 teaspoon turmeric
- 1/2 teaspoon cayenne pepper (adjust for spice preference)
- Salt and pepper to taste
- 2 tablespoons olive oil
- Fresh cilantro, chopped (for garnish)
- Brown rice or quinoa (for serving)

Directions:

1. **Prepare Chickpeas:** If using dried chickpeas, soak them overnight in water. Drain and rinse before use. If using canned chickpeas, make sure to rinse and drain them.
2. **Cook Sweet Potatoes:** Peel and dice sweet potatoes into bite-sized pieces. Steam or boil them until just tender. Set aside.
3. **Sauté Aromatics:** In a large pan, heat olive oil over medium heat. Add chopped onions and sauté until translucent. Add minced garlic and grated ginger, cooking for an additional 1-2 minutes.
4. **Spice it Up:** Stir in curry powder, cumin, coriander, turmeric, cayenne pepper, salt, and pepper. Cook the spices for 2-3 minutes to release their flavors.
5. **Add Tomatoes and Coconut Milk:** Pour in diced tomatoes (with juices) and coconut milk. Stir well to combine. Simmer for 5 minutes to allow the flavors to meld.
6. **Combine Chickpeas and Sweet Potatoes:** Add chickpeas and cooked sweet potatoes to the curry mixture. Stir gently to coat them with the sauce. Simmer for an additional 10-15 minutes until everything is heated through.
7. **Adjust Seasoning:** Taste and adjust salt and pepper as needed. If you prefer a thinner consistency, you can add a bit of vegetable broth or water.
8. **Serve:** Serve the chickpea and sweet potato curry over brown rice or quinoa. Garnish with chopped cilantro.

Nutritional Information per serving: Calories: ~400 kcal, Protein: ~10g, Fat: ~15g, Carbohydrates: ~55g, Fiber: ~12g

Broccoli and Cheese Stuffed Baked Potatoes

Ingredients:

- 4 medium-sized russet potatoes
- 2 cups broccoli florets, steamed
- 1 cup shredded reduced-fat cheddar cheese
- 1/2 cup low-fat Greek yogurt
- 2 green onions, finely chopped
- 2 cloves garlic, minced
- 1 tablespoon olive oil
- Salt and pepper to taste

Directions:

1. **Preheat the Oven:** Preheat your oven to 400°F (200°C).

2. **Prepare Potatoes:** Wash and scrub the potatoes thoroughly. Pierce them with a fork a few times to allow steam to escape during baking.

3. **Bake Potatoes:** Place the potatoes directly on the oven rack and bake for about 45-60 minutes or until tender. The exact time depends on the size of your potatoes.

4. **Prepare Filling:** In a skillet, heat olive oil over medium heat. Add minced garlic and sauté for a minute until fragrant. Add steamed broccoli florets and cook for an additional 2-3 minutes. Season with salt and pepper.

5. **Scoop Potatoes:** Once the potatoes are baked and cooled slightly, cut a slit lengthwise on the top of each potato. Scoop out the flesh, leaving a thin layer to support the skin.

6. **Make Filling:** In a bowl, mash the scooped potato flesh. Mix in Greek yogurt, shredded cheddar cheese, sautéed broccoli, and green onions. Season with salt and pepper to taste.

7. **Stuff Potatoes:** Spoon the broccoli and cheese mixture back into the potato shells, distributing it evenly among the potatoes.

8. **Bake Again:** Place the stuffed potatoes on a baking sheet and bake for an additional 15-20 minutes or until the cheese is melted and bubbly.

9. **Serve:** Remove from the oven and let them cool for a few minutes. Serve warm, garnished with extra green onions if desired.

Nutritional Information per serving: Calories: ~300, Protein: ~12g, Carbohydrates: ~50g, Fat: ~7g, Fiber: ~7g

MEAL PLANS

Day 1:
Breakfast: Oatmeal with Berries
Lunch: Grilled Salmon with Quinoa and Steamed Vegetables
Snack: Greek Yogurt with Berries
Dinner: Baked Chicken Breast with Sweet Potato and Broccoli

Day 2:
Breakfast: Greek Yogurt Parfait with Honey and Nuts
Lunch: Vegetarian Stir-Fry with Tofu and Mixed Vegetables
Snack: Nut Mix
Dinner: Mushroom and Spinach Quiche with Whole Grain Crust

Day 3:
Breakfast: Avocado Toast with Whole Grain Bread
Lunch: Turkey and Vegetable Skewers with Quinoa Salad
Snack: Dark Chocolate-Dipped Strawberries
Dinner: Baked Cod with Asparagus and Lemon

Day 4:
Breakfast: Smoothie Bowl with Spinach and Banana
Lunch: Chickpea and Vegetable Curry with Brown Rice
Snack: Hummus and Whole Grain Crackers
Dinner: Lean Beef Stir-Fry with Bok Choy and Quinoa

Day 5:
Breakfast: Vegetable Omelette
Lunch: Eggplant and Lentil Moussaka
Snack: Guacamole with Veggie Sticks
Dinner: Shrimp and Zucchini Noodles with Pesto

Day 6:
Breakfast: Quinoa Breakfast Bowl with Sliced Fruits
Lunch: Caprese Skewers
Snack: Roasted Chickpeas
Dinner: Greek Salad with Grilled Chicken

Day 7:
Breakfast: Chia Seed Pudding with Fruit
Lunch: Veggie Sushi Rolls
Snack: Baked Apples with Cinnamon and Walnuts
Dinner: Stuffed Bell Peppers with Lean Ground Turkey

CUSTOMIZING FOR INDIVIDUAL NEEDS

1. **Personal Preferences:** Modify recipes depending on personal taste preferences. For instance, if someone prefers vegetarian choices, substitute meat-based foods with plant-based alternatives high in protein.

2. **Caloric Requirements:** Adjust serving sizes to fit individual caloric demands. This is vital for people striving for weight control. Consulting with a dietician may assist identify proper calorie amounts?

3. **Food Allergies or Sensitivities:** Take into consideration any food allergies or sensitivities. Substitute items to satisfy dietary restrictions while creating a balanced and liver-friendly dinner.

4. **Medical issues:** Consider any concurrent medical issues. Individuals with illnesses like diabetes may need to watch carbohydrate consumption. Collaborate with healthcare specialists to adjust the food plan properly.

5. **Cultural Influences:** Integrate cultural preferences into the food plan. Adapt recipes to correspond with varied culinary traditions, offering a more pleasurable and sustainable approach to a liver-friendly diet.

6. **Time limits:** Streamline recipes depending on time limits. Opt for simpler preparations on hectic days, and create bigger portions for handy leftovers.

7. **Nutritional objectives:** Align the food plan with particular nutritional objectives. If there's a requirement for additional fiber or particular vitamins, concentrate on ingesting meals that support those aims.

8. **Hydration:** Emphasize the significance of hydration. Encourage the consumption of water throughout the day and explore herbal teas as delicious alternatives.

9. **Monitoring Progress:** Regularly assess progress and change the food plan as required. This might require reassessing dietary needs, changing recipes, or getting extra help from healthcare specialists.

10. **Customized Wellness strategy:** Develop a comprehensive, customized wellness strategy. Beyond diet, add lifestyle aspects such as stress management and physical exercise, acknowledging their influence on liver health.

Remember, customization is crucial in building a sustainable and successful strategy to controlling fatty liver. Consulting with a trained dietician or healthcare expert ensures that individual requirements are taken into consideration, supporting a targeted and effective path toward liver health.

LIFESTYLE TIPS

1. **Aerobic Exercise:** Engage in frequent aerobic activities such as brisk walking, running, cycling, or swimming. These exercises help burn calories, promote weight reduction, and increase insulin sensitivity, all useful for controlling fatty liver.

2. **Strength Training:** Incorporate strength training routines to improve muscular mass. Increased muscle mass may boost metabolism and aid to overall weight control.

3. **Interval Training:** Include interval training in your regimen. Alternating between high-intensity and lower-intensity exercise has proved to be useful in enhancing metabolic health and lowering liver fat.

4. **Consistency is Key:** Establish a regular workout plan. Aim for at least 150 minutes of moderate-intensity aerobic activity each week, coupled with strength training activities at least twice a week.

5. **Gradual Progression:** Start softly and steadily raise the intensity and length of your exercises. Gradual progression decreases the danger of damage and makes it more sustainable over time.

6. **Choose Enjoyable Activities:** Select workouts you love to boost adherence. Whether it's dancing, hiking, or playing a sport, choosing things you enjoy makes it more likely that you'll continue to your workout program.

7. **Post-Meal Walks:** Incorporate brief walks after meals. Research reveals that post-meal walks may help manage blood sugar levels and enhance insulin sensitivity, which is advantageous for persons with fatty liver.

8. **Flexibility and Balance Exercises:** Include flexibility and balance exercises. Activities like yoga or tai chi may increase general physical well-being and complement cardio and strength training.

9. **Stay Hydrated:** Maintain appropriate hydration throughout activity. Water is necessary for general health and assists in several physiological functions, including the metabolism of fat.

10. **Speak with Healthcare specialists:** Before beginning a new fitness plan, particularly for persons with current health concerns, speak with healthcare specialists. They may give recommendations on acceptable activities and assist guarantee safety.

Regular physical exercise has a critical role in treating fatty liver by encouraging weight reduction, boosting insulin sensitivity, and strengthening overall metabolic health. Tailoring exercise regimens to individual interests and ability levels leads to a sustainable and pleasurable approach to fitness and liver health.

STRESS MANAGEMENT FOR FATTY LIVER

1. **Mindfulness Meditation:** Practice mindfulness meditation to develop awareness and minimize stress. Mindful breathing and meditation practices may significantly improve mental well-being and perhaps lead to better liver function.

2. **Yoga and Relaxation methods:** Engage in yoga or other relaxation methods. Gentle stretching, deep breathing, and relaxation positions may help ease tension and generate a feeling of peace.

3. **Frequent Exercise:** Incorporate frequent physical exercise into your regimen. Exercise is not only helpful for the body but also functions as a stress reliever, generating endorphins that boost mood.

4. **Time Management:** Organize and prioritize activities to manage time efficiently. Having a planned routine helps lessen feelings of overload and aid to stress reduction.

5. **Social Support:** Build a support network. Share concerns with friends, family, or a support group. Social ties give emotional support and may be a significant resource in times of stress.

6. **Good Sleep Habits:** Prioritize good sleep. Establish a consistent sleep regimen and establish a pleasant sleep environment. Quality sleep is vital for stress management and general well-being.

7. **Journaling:** Keep a stress diary to identify stresses and create ways for coping. Writing down ideas and emotions may be a helpful approach to handle stresses.

8. **Limit Stimulants:** Limit the consumption of stimulants like coffee and nicotine, particularly in the evening. These chemicals may lead to increased stress and alter sleep habits.

9. **Mindful Eating:** Practice mindful eating. Paying attention to the tastes, flavors, and textures of food may build a healthy connection with eating and prevent stress-related emotional eating.

10. **Professional help:** Seek professional help if required. Counselors, therapists, or support groups may give ways for dealing with stress and treating its underlying causes.

Stress management is critical for patients with fatty liver, since prolonged stress may damage liver function. Integrating these tactics into everyday life may assist not just to stress reduction but also to the general well-being of both the mind and the liver. It's crucial to personalize stress management approaches to individual tastes and demands. If pressures continue or become unbearable, obtaining help from healthcare specialists is advised.

SLEEP AND ITS IMPACT ON FATTY LIVER

1. **Sleep Duration**: - Aim for 7-9 hours of excellent sleep every night. Inadequate sleep has been connected with insulin resistance, which may contribute to the development and progression of fatty liver.

2. **Regular Sleep routine:** Maintain a regular sleep routine. Going to bed and getting up at the same time each day helps regulate the body's internal clock, supporting greater sleep quality.

3. **Sleep Hygiene:** Establish appropriate sleep hygiene routines. Create a calming evening ritual, keep the bedroom dark and cool, and minimize exposure to electronics before bedtime to increase the quality of sleep.

4. **Sleep Apnea Management:** Address sleep apnea if present. Sleep apnea has been associated to an increased risk of non-alcoholic fatty liver disease (NAFLD). Treatment of sleep apnea, such as utilizing a continuous positive airway pressure (CPAP) device, may significantly improve liver function.

5. **Circadian cycle Alignment:** Align activities with the body's circadian cycle. This includes exposure to natural light in the morning, which helps regulate the sleep-wake cycle and improves general circadian health.

6. **Avoid Late-Night Eating:** Avoid heavy or big meals close to sleep. Late-night eating may interfere with digestion and impair sleep, possibly influencing metabolic processes connected to fatty liver.

7. **Limit Caffeine and Alcohol:** Limit caffeine and alcohol consumption, particularly in the hours preceding up to sleep. Both medications may interfere with sleep quality and disturb the body's normal sleep-wake cycle.

8. **Exercise Regularly:** Engage in regular physical activity, but avoid severe exercise close to sleep. Regular exercise has been linked to improved sleep, but timing is key to minimize any disturbances.

9. **Stress Management:** Manage stress to encourage peaceful sleep. Stress and poor sleep are interrelated, and good stress management may significantly improve sleep quality.

10. **Seek Professional help:** If sleep issues continue, consider getting professional help. Sleep problems or persistent insomnia may need examination and assistance from healthcare specialists.

Prioritizing excellent sleep hygiene and resolving sleep-related concerns may help to overall metabolic health and may have a favorable influence on the prevention and treatment of fatty liver. Individuals having recurrent sleep issues should speak with healthcare specialists for a full examination and suitable therapies.

CONCLUSION

In closing the "Fatty Liver Recipes Cookbook," it's apparent that the road toward liver health entails more than simply a collection of recipes—it's a comprehensive approach to feeding the body and fostering overall well-being. The cookbook acts as a guide, presenting a varied selection of tasty and nutritionally balanced dishes targeted to benefit those managing or avoiding fatty liver disease.

Through the careful selection of ingredients and conscious consideration of macronutrients and micronutrients, the cookbook allows readers to make educated decisions that contribute to liver health. The introduction of a range of tastes, textures, and culinary styles ensures that adopting a liver-friendly diet stays a fun and lasting lifestyle adjustment.

Beyond the kitchen, the cookbook highlights the role of lifestyle factors in controlling fatty liver. From stress management and regular exercise to appropriate sleep, the recipes are complimented with information on cultivating a balanced and health-promoting lifestyle.

As readers explore the pages of the "Fatty Liver Recipes Cookbook," they go on a gastronomic adventure that stretches well beyond flavor alone. It is a path toward better well-being, inspired by the idea that dietary choices and lifestyle practices play vital roles in promoting liver health. By accepting the ideas contained in this cookbook, people may take proactive steps toward a healthy future, appreciating not only the pleasures of each meal but also the delight of feeding their bodies from inside.

In concluding, may the "Fatty Liver Recipes Cookbook" encourage a continual commitment to mindful eating, an appreciation of varied and healthy foods, and a persistent devotion to overall health?

FREQUENTLY ASKED QUESTIONS

Why a cookbook is primarily focused on fatty liver dishes important?
Fatty liver disease demands a detailed nutritional strategy. This cookbook is geared to give meals high in nutrients that promote liver health, making it a helpful resource for anyone treating or avoiding fatty liver.

Are the dishes in this cookbook acceptable for all dietary preferences?
Yes, the cookbook includes a range of.

How may these recipes aid someone with non-alcoholic fatty liver disease (NAFLD)?
The recipes concentrate on complete, nutrient-dense meals proven to enhance liver function. Incorporating these dishes into a balanced diet may benefit in controlling NAFLD by supporting weight management, lowering inflammation, and enhancing overall liver function.

Can these meals be part of a weight control strategy for patients with fatty liver?
Absolutely. The meals stress whole foods, lean proteins, and healthy fats, making them excellent for anyone wanting to control or reduce weight. Combined with a healthy lifestyle, these meals add to a complete approach to weight control.

How can this cookbook be used in combination with medical advice for fatty liver management?
While the cookbook gives helpful nutritional guidelines, it's crucial to check with healthcare specialists for tailored counsel. The recipes may complement medical suggestions, giving a practical and entertaining approach to execute nutritional modifications.

Are there recipes suited for persons with time restrictions or hectic schedules?
Yes, the cookbook features dishes that adapt to varied time restrictions. Quick and simple solutions are available, ensuring that those with hectic schedules may still enjoy nutritional, liver-friendly meals without losing flavor or health benefits.

Can the cookbook assist with meal planning for those with fatty liver?
Certainly. The cookbook contains a varied selection of dishes for breakfast, lunch, supper, snacks, and desserts. Readers may use these recipes as a basis for building well-rounded, liver-friendly meal plans that correspond with their interests and dietary requirements.

How can the dishes in the cookbook assist to a sustainable and satisfying dietary change?
The cookbook promotes tastes, textures, and a diversity of ingredients to make liver-friendly eating fun. By including different and delectable meals, it fosters a sustainable approach to dietary changes, promoting a good and long-lasting influence on overall health.

Are there tools or recommendations available for persons shifting to a liver-friendly diet?
Yes, the cookbook contains tools and ideas for folks switching to a liver-friendly diet. This contains information on food replacements, culinary methods, and practical recommendations for making the transition simpler and more pleasurable.

How many readers submit comments or seek further information connected to the cookbook?
Readers may find contact information inside the cookbook for submitting comments or requesting further information. Whether its inquiries about particular recipes or requests for further assistance, the objective is to encourage folks on their road to improved liver health.

GLOSSARY

1. **Fatty Liver Disease:** A disorder defined by the buildup of fat in liver cells, generally related with lifestyle factors such as obesity and poor dietary choices.

2. **NAFLD (Non-Alcoholic Fatty Liver Disease):** A kind of fatty liver disease not induced by alcohol usage, including a spectrum of disorders from basic fatty liver to non-alcoholic steatohepatitis (NASH).

3. **Omega-3 Fatty Acids:** Essential fatty acids present in some fish, flaxseeds, and walnuts, recognized for their anti-inflammatory qualities.

4. **Insulin Resistance:** A condition where cells fail to react efficiently to insulin, resulting to high blood sugar levels; a factor in the development of fatty liver.

5. **Antioxidants:** Compounds in foods like berries and leafy greens that help counteract oxidative stress and inflammation in the body.

6. **Lean Proteins:** Protein foods with minimal fat content, such as chicken, fish, tofu, and lentils.

7. **Whole Grains:** Grains that retain all portions of the seed, giving additional nutrients and fiber; examples include quinoa, brown rice, and whole wheat.

8. **Hydration:** Maintaining enough water consumption to improve general health, including liver function.

9. **Stress Management:** Techniques and behaviors aimed at lowering stress, which might impair liver health.

10. **Circadian Rhythm:** The body's inherent internal clock that controls sleep-wake cycles and numerous physiological activities.

11. **Macronutrients:** Essential nutrients necessary by the body in relatively significant quantities, including carbs, proteins, and lipids.

12. **Micronutrients:** Essential nutrients required in lower quantities, such as vitamins and minerals.

13. **Inflammation:** The body's reaction to damage or infection, commonly connected to fatty liver and other chronic disorders.

14. **Metabolism:** The process by which the body turns food into energy and carries out numerous physiological activities.

15. **Portion Control:** Managing the quantity of food ingested in a single sitting to limit calorie intake.

16. **Meal Planning:** Strategically planning meals to promote a balanced and healthy diet.

17. **Mindful Eating:** Paying attention to the sensory experience of eating, establishing a healthy connection with food.

18. **Dietary Fiber:** The indigestible portion of plant foods that assists un digestion and leads to a sensation of fullness.

19. **Probiotics:** Beneficial bacteria that improve gut health, found in fermented foods like yogurt and kefir.

20. **Hepatic Steatosis:** Another word for fatty liver, characterized by the buildup of fat in liver cells.

21. **BMI (Body Mass Index):** A measure of body fat based on height and weight, typically used to determine weight status.

22. **Glucose:** A form of sugar that acts as the body's principal source of energy.

23. **Trans Fats:** Artificially manufactured fats present in certain processed foods, known to lead to inflammation and liver disorders.

24. **Meal Prep:** Planning and preparing meals in advance to support healthy eating habits.

25. **Nutrient-Dense Foods:** Foods that give a high number of nutrients compared to their calorie content.

26. **Liver Function Tests:** Blood tests that measure the health and function of the liver by measuring particular enzymes and proteins.